The Shaolin Martial Arts

The Spirit of the
Five Animals

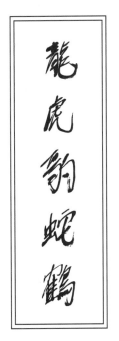

The Shaolin Martial Arts

The Spirit of the Five Animals

Tak Wah Eng

Creative Art Director: Tak Wah Eng
Transcription: Tak Wah Eng
Graphic Designer: Jason Ng
Photographers: Kelly Fung, Marc Waithe, Edwin Wu
Writers: Hotay Ma and Jason Ng
Contributors: Allen Chan, Vincent Lai,
            Gary Ma and the students of the
            Tak Wah Shaolin Kung Fu Club.

Dedicated to the many students
that devote themselves
to martial arts.

Contents

Steps

A thousand mile road begins with one step.
Even masters were once students.
If you take the first step, you will get there.

Time

Do not regret what has past.
One must not be too eager for what is to come.
Have health and benefit from the moment.
Let go of yesterday and start brand new,
Because time is always passing.
Embrace the moment,
Before it becomes lost.

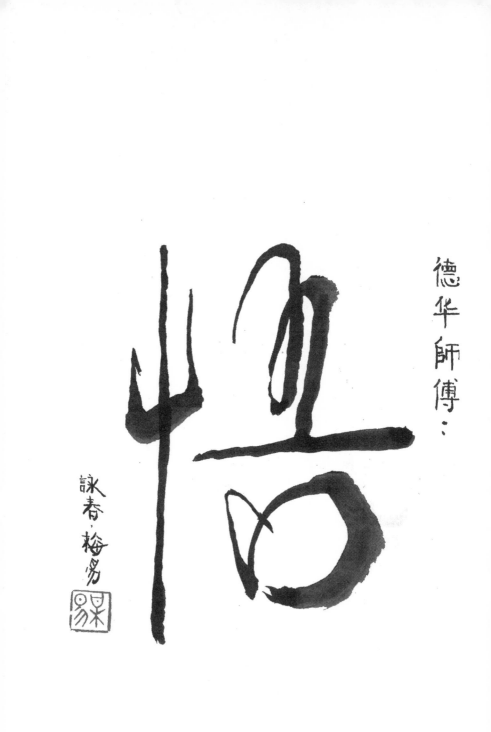

德华師傅：

詠春·梅易

During the Dynastic period, there lived an Emperor in China who had developed his country into a prosperous one through his many deeds and just ruling. This Emperor had been the giving and good spirit that aided his people from poverty and sickness. As it is natural, one who gives so much sometimes expect something more in return. The Emperor through his generosity seeked the Zen Master known as Dat Mo for his personal advisory. Dat Mo was well-known throughout China and gained a reputation among the people as a wise and knowledgeable man.

As the great Zen Master entered the halls of the palace, he was greeted by the guards and escorted into the Emperor's private chambers. It is there that the Emperor imposed many questions for Dat Mo. Dat Mo advised him in governmental as well as personal issues. He would ask what would benefit him more in his actions and how he could better serve himself for the country. The Emperor also expressed that he deserved the greatest of riches and the most beautiful bride he was currently seeking. He expressed that he had done a great amount for his country and therefore should be rewarded justly. The Zen Master looked into the Emperor's eyes and saw the reflection of his spirit. Although a good man, he seeked rewards for his valor and saw this within the Emperor. Dat Mo replied that the idea of Zen is to focus on the act itself.

The actions of the Emperor had given a great reward that he neglected to see. The people of his country no longer suffered as harshly as they did before. There is a strong bond formed by the people towards the Emperor that sits here before the Zen Master. Expecting a reward for one's action is not the proper way of seeing things. It is within the knowledge of the action itself and nothing else is there a true understanding. Focus on the action and not the reward. Focus on the man that has given so much wealth, prosperity and a willingness to share knowledge in educating the people. It is during this time that the Emperor began to understand the idea of the action itself.

During the creation of this book I had been able to talk to Sifu Tak Wah Eng. I had known that he had contributed to teaching to many students and written several books on the subject of martial arts. He had also contributed in many workshops and session to educate the people more about the world of martial arts. He carried with his teaching a certain energy and enthusiasm that each person feels when speaking to him. He has been awarded many honors in the martial arts world. So it was then that I asked him if he has done such a large amount to help others then he should be expecting things back from those students. Sifu Eng then answered in his calm way of explaining, that he does this to help all his students to enrich their knowledge of martial arts and to become successful in their lives. He applies this ideology towards his life and is simply showing others how to do so themselves. Along the way his students may be able to benefit not just from martial arts but also towards their lives. Sifu Tak believes that his students should reflect upon their daily actions but also to move ahead. He then said something that I have remembered for the longest time. He said "All my students become my teacher because they have so much to learn and so do I." He continued stating that it is through his students and himself and a large amount of focus that this book has come into fruition. I understand that to me now that it is a joint effort and diligence that such a project as this book was possible. The gathering of different minds and personality helped in creating this book in order to pass on to other students. Near the end of the meeting he described his work in a very interesting way. He stated that his work was "... A road or a highway that is to be traveled on in the future." His work was a building block that continued to stretch across the way. This road he believes is a continuation of his knowledge that will be able to lead other students in the future towards the same path. It is through this realization about his work that he does not ask for anything in return. He believes that his action at the present time is an accomplishment. The benefit that his students gain through his teaching is the reward within itself.

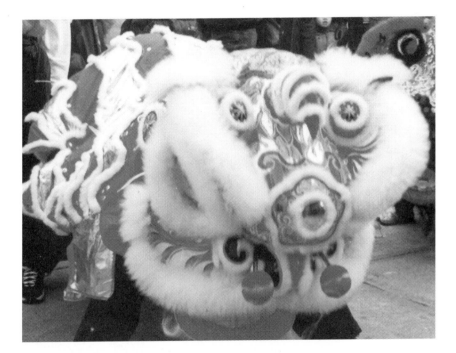

Foreword

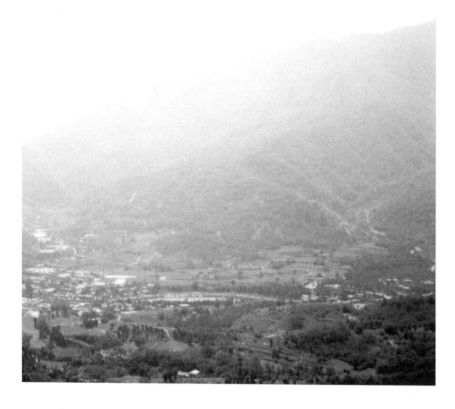

When I first met Sifu Tak Wah Eng many years ago I had already been a practitioner of several different styles of martial arts. I was, however, in an extremely distressed mental state since a knee injury had taken such a toll on me. On many mornings just getting out of bed and standing up without excruciating pain was a challenge. What was worse was that I had worked as an anesthesiologist and knew the wonderful outcome that "modern medicine" (and the surgeon's cold steel blade) would offer me. It was not for any belief in Chi Kung or Kung Fu's curative aspect which drew me towards him. I simply did not know enough about this form of martial arts at the time to make any critical judgement about it. Yet, I sensed an inner calmness as well as an extremely powerful presence in this unassuming man; Someone not motivated by material gain but one who lives and breathes the walk and talk of Kung Fu (which literally means a dedicated study over a long period of time).

Having a curious nature and a love for Eastern philosophy and medicine, I had been drawn to the art and science of acupuncture and Chinese medicine many years ago and certainly many years before the hordes of Western trained doctors began flocking to it (and unfortunately reducing it to another medical treatment protocol and billing code). Serving as the Dean and Medical Director of the University of Natural Medicine in Santa Fe, New Mexico, I taught courses in Eastern medicine, acupuncture, pain management, and "Chi."

Even though I "understood" what Chi was (this is just
scratching the surface for one must experience it) and my students
were awed by my scientific explanation of it, deep down in my heart
I knew that I never experienced its power. Sure, I had seen some
what appeared to be a fantastic demonstration of it by "masters."
In fact, right at that time I joined a large group in a very
commercialized trip to the Shaolin Temple in China. Master
Eng was one of the teachers in the group. When he took me
and several of his top students to the inner sanctum of the temple
(where the true monks train and meditate) and introduced me
to the real masters and not the "Disneyland" version I knew.
This area was, of course, off limits to the scores of other people
on the trip.

It was at this point that I called Master Eng and asked him
if he would train me. He told me to come in and we sat, and had
some tea (just like in the old tradition of teacher and student).
During this time he received two phone calls and from what
I heard in the other room, he actually threw away potential
business by telling these people that he did not take on new students.
I instinctively knew that this was the real deal. I knew that my search
for the master teacher had come to an end. He would become
the doctor's doctor (in the true Shaolin sense). He first watched
me perform some movements and gave me the Chi Kung classic
"The Eight Pieces of Silk" to practice.

As I mastered this, the homework became tougher and
tougher. I began to actually experience the sensation of Chi and harn-
essed its amazing power. The real validation came on a medical
trip to Russia. While I was lecturing alongside Russia's top scient-
ists, one person wanted to "measure my Chi" (or life energy).
He hooked me up to a "Kirlian Photography" machine and
within minutes it printed out in full color, a complete proj-
ection of my aura or bioelectrical energy field. The jet lag,
the many days of travel, and the lecturing without rest had taken its

toll. It was weak. I asked the head doctor if I may be excused and do Chi Kung for five to ten minutes and have it measured again. They shrugged and said sure. When it was measured the results blew them away and left them speechless to say the least. I have since taught them the form and they are still in contact with me as students.

This is but one small example of the benefits of my practice. It has helped me get through some of the toughest personal challenges of my life. In fact, I have completed a book on the medical benefits of Chi Kung so that other people may share its knowledge and wisdom. I am blessed to have met this great master and human being. Master Eng has an uncanny ability to look into and read the spirit of people (medical doctors are still fumbling with this one!) Thus, I would never know what I would be getting myself into when I arrived for class (a hard core fighting lesson, some "Soft Chi Kung," Buddhist spiritual guidance, or just plain old-fashion psychotherapy.) I guess this is the true Kung Fu of life.

Bill Akpinar, DDS, MD
Dean and Medical Director
University of Natural Medicine

Introduction

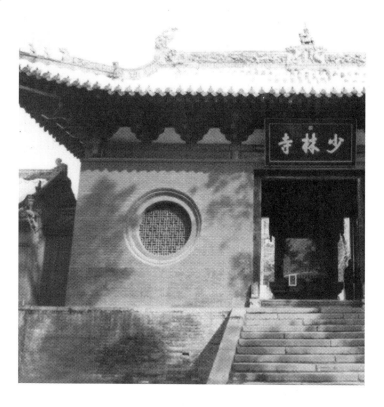

Those that have decided to pick up this book range between novice to experts. This book goes through the basic fundamentals and the advanced forms that are encompassed within the Five Animals System. The philosophy and ideology of martial arts is also included. This book is separated into different aspects of the mind and the body. It is through a balance between both aspects can an individual benefit from martial arts.

Martial arts is a self discovery of the abilities each individual has inherent within themselves. The human body is capable of miraculous things. Shaolin monks have trained their whole lives to develop their body and mind. There is a structured system within martial arts, however, there is also a place for self expression, hence the word art.

People bring their own personal experiences, beliefs, and attitudes that make each individual unique. The person defines the martial arts. A teacher can teach the basic fundamentals of a style or system, but at some point the teacher has taught everything. This is where the student is left to discover and define their own martial arts style. In establishing a strong foundation the person has then the freedom to explore. By practicing your movements, you have begun your own personal journey to defining your own martial arts.

Testimonials

德华师傅：

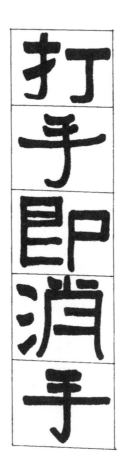

詠春·检易

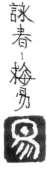

Life is the interaction of people and the experiences and memories they share with each other. When people share these things together it bonds them. An individual can affect many people with their personal perspective and philosophy. Sifu Tak Wah Eng has met many people from his travels through his lifelong commitment towards martial arts. These area handful of testimonials from many of Sifu Eng's teachers and students. They describe the scope of how one person's teachings have affected their own personal lives. Through these testimonials the reader will gain an understanding to how martial arts and a different perspective in approaching things can change their lives permanently.

Several years ago, my martial arts instructor invited me to one of his classes with Master Tak Wah Eng. I could tell that there was something different about the way Master Eng taught. He had something that my previous instructors were missing. I was not really sure exactly what it was until I got to know him better, but it was the spiritual side of the martial arts that Master Eng possessed.

I had not realized that I had only been taught the physical side of the martial arts, which may be great in a self defense situation, but is not that useful in my everyday life. Most people will continue their entire lives without ever having to defend themselves physically, but everyone has internal battles to fight.

While Master Tak Wah Eng is a skilled martial artist with a tremendous knowledge of Shaolin Kung Fu, it is his inner strength and peaceful spirit that I admire the most.

Master Brian Hanson
7th Dan Kempo Instructor
Martial Arts Training Center
Cheshire, CT

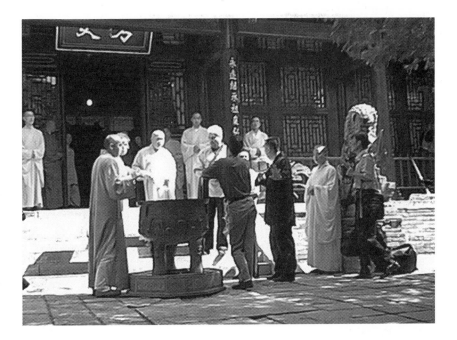

I was first introduced to Grand Master Tak Wah Eng during a black belt instruction morning workout in Connecticut, approximately ten years ago. This introduction was made possible by my teacher, Grandmaster Stephen B. DeMasco, for whom I will always be grateful for giving me this opportunity. As I enthusiastically waited in anticipation of this meeting, my expectations were very high. After all, this was my teacher's teacher. Needless to say, he exceeded my expectations. During the following years to come, my meetings became more frequent and memorable as I began to learn from Grandmaster Tak Wah Eng himself.

What truly stands out in my mind is how blessed I felt to have the opportunity to train with an extraordinary martial artist, and to have him as a mentor. Through Grandmaster Eng's teachings, I learned many important lessons which have transcended how I live my professional and personal life and achieve goals in those areas. One lesson in particular that came to me while training, where I was striving for perfection, was the notion that it was hard to achieve a level of perfection, so I said to myself, "the day you think you are good enough is the day you stop getting better." This life motto has helped me realize that there really is no such thing as perfection; just levels of mastery. There are many martial artists who once achieve mastery, do not further try to seek out ways to improve themselves, as opposed to Grandmaster Tak Wah Eng who constantly trains, focuses on self improvement, and personally teaches his students to respect the same principles. To see a man with extraordinary levels of martial arts ability, train in the hope that he will still work towards improving himself both physically and mentally, gives me great motivation and determination to improve myself on a daily basis. After each training session I feel invigorated, especially after being up long hours as a result of my overwhelming schedule juggling a family and two careers in law enforcement and martial arts instruction. Grandmaster Tak Wah Eng is one of the most talented martial artists that I have personally had the honor to train under. He is a humble, patient, philosophical, and practical man.

Grandmaster Tak Wah Eng has helped me become a better instructor, and has inspired me to reach certain physical goals that I thought were unattainable especially later in life. As I was getting older, I was not getting slower. Instead I was getting faster and stronger. At all phases of training, I witnessed great changes in my own abilities; change that surpassed my own expectations.

On another note, we were able to share great experiences when we were in China at the Shaolin Temple. Training together on the ancient grounds, walking the Great Wall of China, and touring the great history of China will always be a lasting memory.

As I make my way into Chinatown each week, I think to myself, what will I learn today? From the moment I leave our training session, I leave feeling inspired in anticipation of our next meeting. Once again, Grandmaster Tak Wah Eng truly is a master teacher, martial artist, and friend. I look forward to our future years in which I will take his teachings and transfer them to my own students in which the cycle will continue once again.

Master Larry S. Boritz
Shaolin Kempo
United Studios of Commack

I had the pleasure of being introduced to Grandmaster Tak Wah Eng about eight years ago. This meeting was through my Kempo master at that time. That is when Grandmaster Eng began teaching me his style of Kung Fu.

Through the years, our bond became stronger. I had the opportunity to travel to China with him and train at the Shaolin Temple. Although we are close in age, I seek his guidance and knowledge. My Kung Fu training is ongoing with Grandmaster Eng and enlightens me at every meeting.

Grandmaster Tak is a true grandmaster in every sense of the title. This publication is a reflection of his intuition and wisdom. I feel it will be an asset to all martial artists. I look forward to many more years of his training and friendship.

Master Richard Spatola
United Studios Virtuous School
Miller Place, NY

Master Tak Wah Eng has been a tremendous inspiration to me both as a martial artist and as a person. I was introduced to his style of martial arts in 1994 when I started training with one of his students. In June of 2000, I had the opportunity to train with him directly on a daily basis while we were in China to visit and train at the Shaolin Temple. It was after this trip that I was afforded the opportunity to start taking private lessons with him. He has guided me both as a martial artist and in the development of martial virtue. His skills as a teacher and as a true martial artist are unsurpassed.

Ross Antisdel
4th Degree Shaolin Kempo Karate
2nd Degree Black Sash in Shaolin Kung Fu

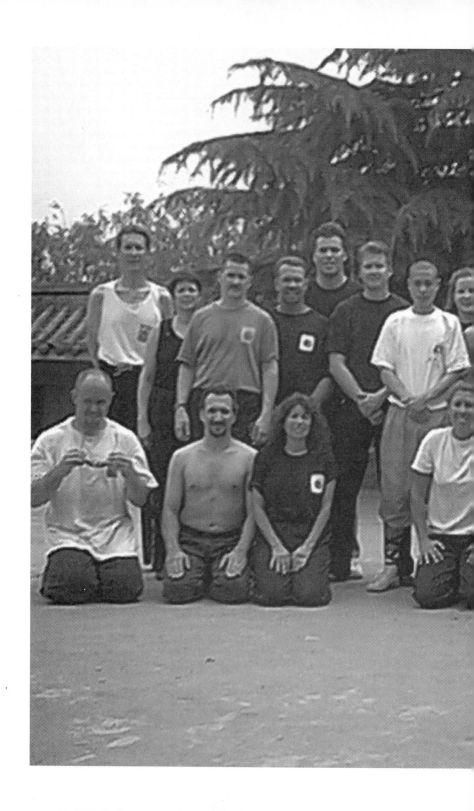

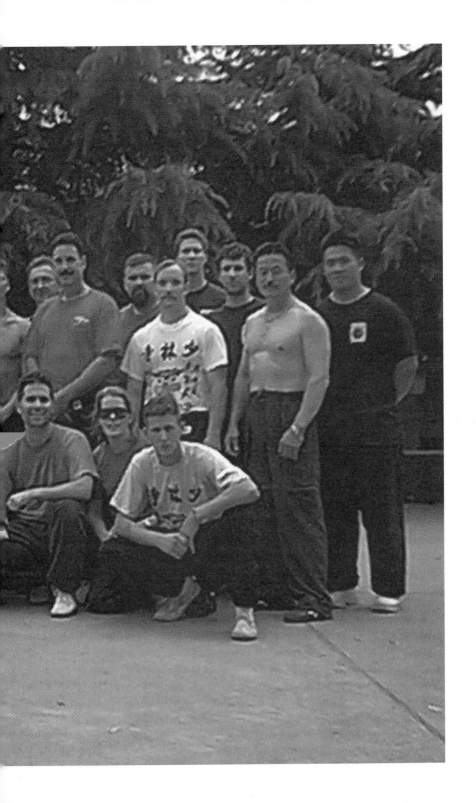

I was first introduced to Master Tak Wah Eng and Five Animals Kung Fu at a clinic that he taught with another master. I had been training in Kempo for a few years and when I saw Master Eng demonstrate the form they were teaching, I immediately noticed a tremendous difference in the way he executed the movements in the form. His movements smooth and graceful, while at the same time powerful and precise. I wanted to learn to move like him. Five years later, I was invited to travel to China and visit the Shaolin Temple. This was also my opportunity to begin training directly with Master Eng. To me, Five Animals Kung Fu is a way to go back in time to when the Shaolin monks first started practicing Kung Fu, mimicking the movements of the tiger, snake, crane, dragon, and leopard. Under Master Eng's guidance I hope to help preserve and pass on the knowledge and spirit of Kung Fu to others.

William K. Hackett
Chief Instructor of Kung Fu and Kempo
Georgetown Martial Arts Center

I would like to share my thoughts of appreciation for my teacher and mentor Master Tak Wah Eng. It is a great honor and pleasure that I have had over a decade of continued training under his guidance. I have found enlightenment and wisdom as well as self cultivation within these many years of training with him.

On July 7, 2000, I had the honor of being elected to represent a delegation from USA to the legendary Shaolin Temple located in Henen Province, Deng Feng County and considered by most the birth place of martial arts.

My audience was the famous Abbot of the Shaolin Temple along with his 30 Shaolin Warrior monks. Our delegation had more than 230 people in attendance. This event was captured and aired by the local as well as Shanghai news. Under the direct guidance of Master Tak Wah Eng, I was elected to perform the rare Shaolin Snake Fist set. I wish to sincerely thank Master Tak Wah Eng for preparing me physically and mentally as well as spiritually for this occasion. In 2002, I was again elected to represent another delegation to China. I was asked to perform the rare Shaolin Black Tiger fist set as taught to me by Sifu Tak Wah Eng. As before, this performance was received well by the Abbot of the Shaolin Temple and his monks. Having had trained in the martial arts for more than twenty years, the years I spent training with Master Tak Wah Eng has been a learning experience that helped me find the way to centering my life. I feel that Master Tak Wah Eng's actual ability to translate the Shaolin philosophy and Chinese culture to an adult or a child is what makes him a great Master of the Martial Arts. His guidance in Zen philosophy as well as his expertise in the Chinese Martial Arts has been priceless to me and my students.

As I continue my journey through the Shaolin Martial Arts as a direct student of Master Tak Wah Eng and as his West Coast-based representative, I can hope to help spread his teaching methods and style of Chinese classical Kung Fu, culture, humbleness, and perseverance. It is with these principles that Master Eng has passed his art onto me as I will do so for my students. He has always been open to share his wealth of knowledge and has been a major role model for me. With respect and admiration, I thank Master Tak Wah Eng for all that he has helped me with. I am sure this publication will be a treasure in all Kung Fu practitioners' libraries.

Giuseppe Aliotta
West Coast Martial Arts Academy
463 Encinitas Blvd
Encinitas, CA 92024

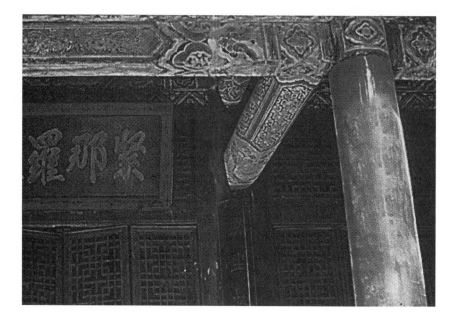

It is with great pleasure to speak of Grandmaster Tak Wah Eng. Grandmaster Eng truly epitomizes the spirit of Shaolin. With nearly a decade of knowing and training with Grandmaster Eng, he has given me the true meaning of honor, respect, and truth. Grandmaster Eng provides numerous years of Shaolin Martial Arts as well as an in-depth knowledge of Zen philosophy. Grandmaster Eng's virtuous teaching ability has guided me to understand the authentic meaning of Kung Fu as well as finding the greatest warrior from within. I truly thank Grandmaster Tak Wah Eng for his time and energy in passing his art on to me. I feel this reading will be a wealth of knowledge to all martial artists.

Sifu Enzo Aliotta, BS, CAT
United Studios Virtuous School
Miller Place, NY

It has been an honor to study the forms of the Shaolin with Sifu Tak Wah Eng. From the first time I saw him teach and demonstrate a form, I was captivated and determined to learn more about this beautiful and powerful art. His movements were the embodiment of balance; yin and yang in motion. This simultaneous power and grace, strength and softness, intensity and peace, was stunning. I made a decision. Whatever it was that enabled a human body to move that way was something I needed in my life.

I would soon learn that Shaolin Kung Fu is far more than a way to move your body. Sifu Eng would teach me that it is a mental focus, an inner peace, and a state of being, united with numerous physical skills born of intense training. Having developed this new interest at age 36, I was afraid that I might be too old to reap the benefits of the ancient art. I still didn't fully understand the concept. Sifu would later clarify that the study and practice of Kung Fu is in fact a journey, not a destination. With each new form comes the opportunity to strengthen your mind, your spirit, and your character, as well as your body. Balance is the key; to avoid excess and focus on improvement and understanding is the challenge. In fact, he reminds me each time I see him that he continues to learn from his students, ever the student himself.

Now, nearly ten years later, I realized that my study of Shaolin Kung Fu has helped me face all the challenges in my life, whether physical, mental or spiritual. The training helps me to balance firmness and kindness, strength and weakness, courage and fear, sorrow and joy, while always seeking to improve and learn. I have learned that it is an honor and a privilege to be "ever the student," no matter what your age or experience. I will be forever grateful to Sifu Tak Wah Eng for the balance and happiness he has brought to my life and to the lives of my children.

Phyllis R. Wasko
Georgetown Martial Arts Center
Redding, CT 06896

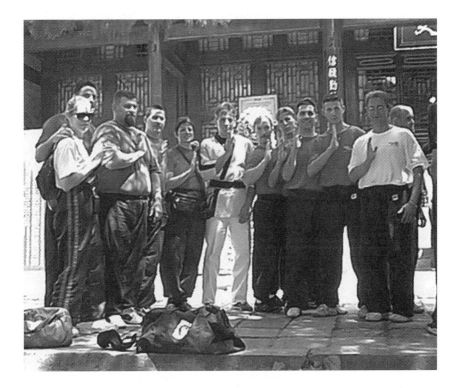

A Trip to China

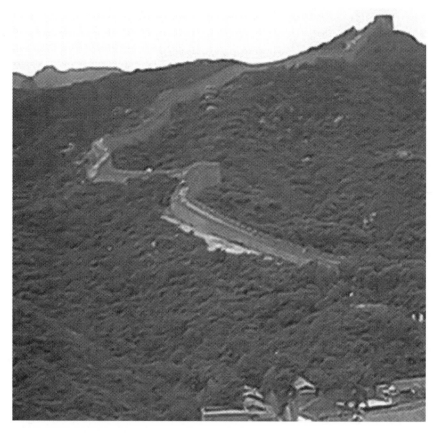

The Great Wall of China spanning across the countryside.

In 2000, Sifu Tak Wah Eng traveled back to China with a group of his students and teachers to experience a rare occasion. Not only were they able to visit the many landmarks of temples and shrines, they had the opportunity to visit the Shaolin Temple. They spent many days experiencing the different environments of the temple and observed the daily ceremonies of the monks. This small group was also able to train with Sifu Tak Wah Eng on these sacred grounds where many believed Kung Fu had originated from.

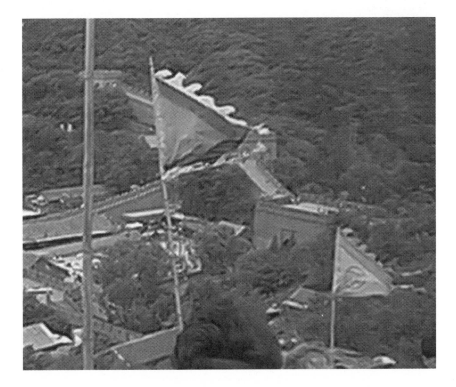

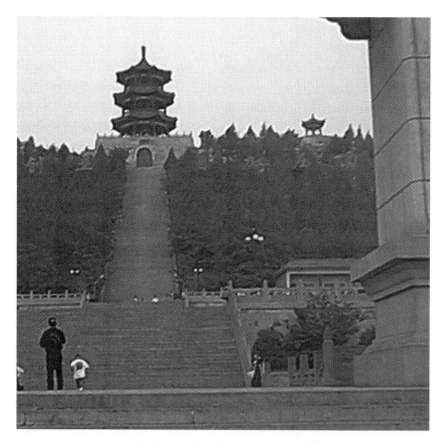

A beautiful shot in front of the Dao Temple in China.

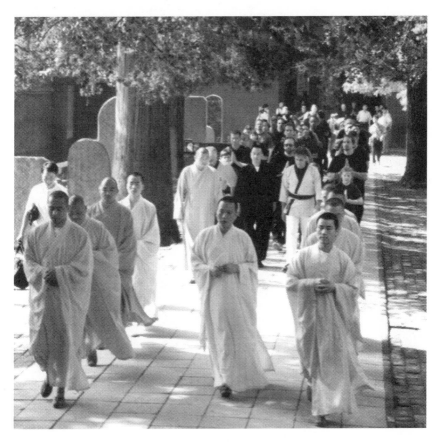

Sifu Tak Wah Eng and his group of students and teachers arrive in China. They are led to the entrance of the Shaolin Temple.

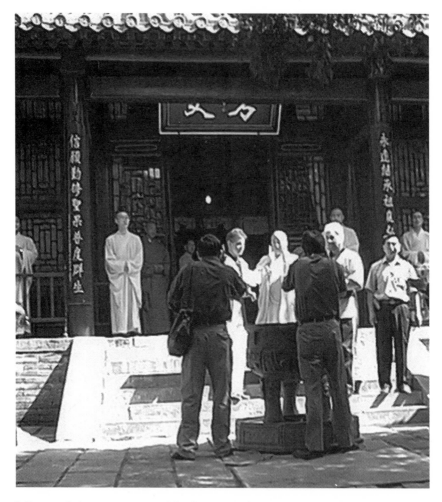

Many of the guests stand in front of the entrance waiting to be received by the Shaolin Abbot.

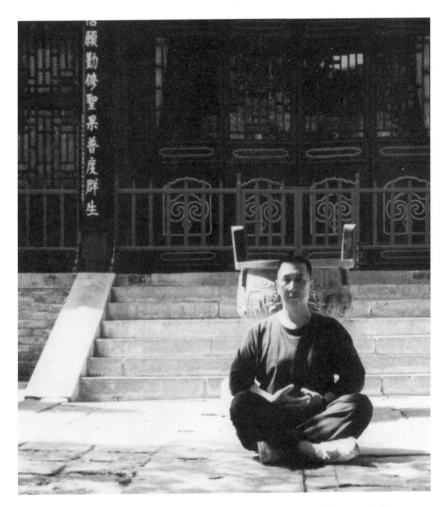

Sifu Tak Wah Eng having a chance to meditate in front of the
Temple in the courtyard.

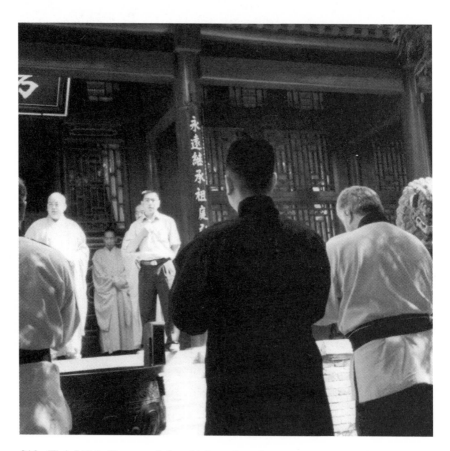

Sifu Tak Wah Eng and the Abbot showing respect to each other.

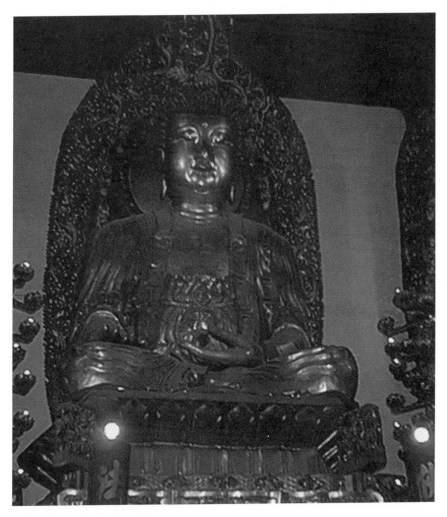

The main Buddha within the Shaolin Temple where the monks gather to perform their ceremonies.

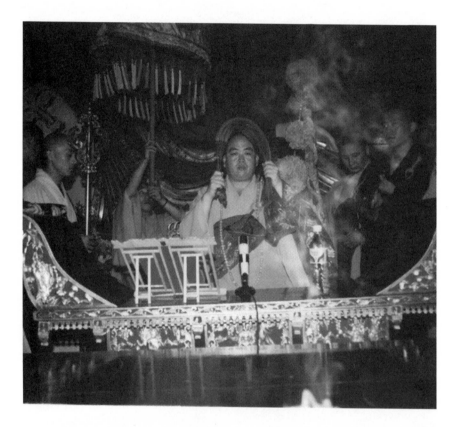

A spiritual ceremony performed by the head Abbot blessing the
monks and visitors.

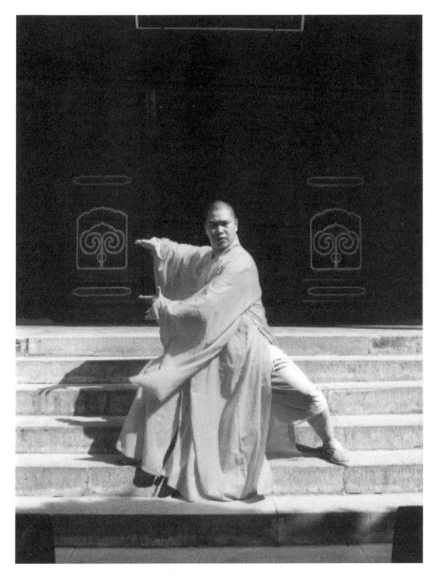

Master Guo Lin at the Shaolin Temple.

Chan and Wu

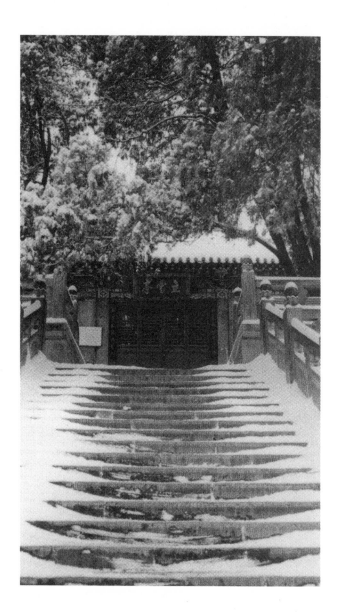

The founding of the Shaolin Temple and its martial arts has been the subject of numerous volumes of books, which include detailed information on religion, combat, excercise, art, music, philosophy, and much more. The Temple is a mystical and spiritual haven enclosed in the mountainous Song area in the heart of China. Throughout history, many people seeking the distinct holiness and enlightenment of Shaolin have traveled many difficult paths to reach it. As an individual we have all faced many obstacles in attaining our goal such as seeking mastery of martial arts and other aspects of our lives. Whether a curious beginner or a seasoned veteran, this book seeks to satisfy a part of the understanding of the vast ideologies and philosophies of the Shaolin Temple. The first subject is the focus on *Chan*.

Chan is the Chinese word originated from the Shaolin teachings to describe the peace and focus involved in a monks pursuit to master their art. The word *Chan* is an idea shared around the world since its beginnings. (This is also known as *Zen* in Japan.) Many other art forms utilize the core features of *Chan* such as Yoga and Tai Chi. In each case, the emphasis is on striving to master the idea of stillness of mind and body.

Chan is a complex idea of different elements of life. It applies to nature and the environment and also towards the mind, body, and soul. It relates to the energy that flows within our bodies and the potentiality of an individual. It deals with the behavior and point of view a person has towards all things that have life. The stillness and focus that is gained within *Chan* can bring forward the realization of self and the people around them. There are many methods of obtaining *Chan* but one must begin with the most basic method and that is the act of breathing.

The first step to gaining and understanding *Chan* in the body and mind is through controlled and natural breathing. Find a quiet place and sit comfortably. Then close your eyes and begin to focus on your breaths. Proper breathing is necessary to gain stillness in the mind and body. Breathing as basic as it is, brings oxygen into the body in order to perform basic and complex life functions. It is taken for granted daily, but setting aside time to sit in a quiet location will bring your mind at ease from the daily stresses. After practicing simple breathing exercises, the mind will begin to focus on the breaths and how the body inhales and exhales. Through continued focus the individual will realize their own being and the consciousness of existence. Once the act of breathing and pure focus can be achieved it can then be applied to daily activities. The obtained focus can provide many benefits internally and externally. This is a simple meditation that will keep the body and mind still for the moment. *Chan* can be precise or general and, at times, centered at different places. *Chan*, in this sense, can have a direct or diverse meaning. A monk once described *Chan* using the following story:

Once there was a person that needed to cross a river. What does he need to cross it? A boat. However, what does the person need from the boat once he has gotten across? He has reached the destination successfully; the boat is redundant and is left behind.

In the end, the boat seems to be worth nothing, but it can also mean everything. The monk could have jumped in and swam across, but by using the boat it would have been the smarter, safer, and drier approach to cross. Shaolin monks have used meditation to keep their *Chan*. Their ability to do incredible feats demonstrates their unrelenting concentration and focus. When studying martial arts, our *Chan* is constantly being contested by influences both internally and externally. The challenge of a Kung Fu practitioner is to keep his concentration despite the difficulties experienced. A mental lapse and the monk will fail in their training.

The endpoint of studying Shaolin martial arts or any other style is subjective to the initial *Chan*. One cannot expect two different novice students of martial arts, with different goals, to end at the same place. In describing this endpoint, it is important to remember that there is no relative superior endpoint, rather, an area in which all consideration one can easily neglect and continue on their path of learning Shaolin martial arts. However, in our main objective to get across the river, one would want a strong and buoyant boat and not a shoddy raft.

The analogy of the boat is but one of the many used by many monks and philosophers of *Chan*. The story of the "Black and White Cloth" gives us a different perspective on *Chan*.

It is natural to adapt, change, and evolve. As a white cloth is put into different colored dyes, the cloth will continually change to a new color. In life, like the cloth, we also change as we go into different situations. We become more vibrant and unique as the breadth of experiences takes us. A black cloth, on the other hand, will never change colors when placed in different dyes. It rejects change and never develops beyond its shady tint.

As we learn in this example, whatever route taken is acceptable; there is no specific formula for a perfect color dye. The key thought raised in this story is the *Chan* used at the very beginning of the process. Students attentive to *Chan* will constantly cleanse themselves of all clutter in their mind. The individual challenges their current knowledge to better understand themselves and the world. Mistakes are bound to happen on the way, but the white cloth is never too dark to become influenced by the positive. Just as one can stray away, one can also excel in their development by following knowledgeable persons who have walked a path similar to their own, a color expert in fabric dyeing.

The idea of *Wu* is much different from *Chan*. It is a more concrete idea. The movements of offense and defense of numerous martial arts styles define *Wu*. Throughout history, countless masters have learned, practiced and expended the art of *Wu*. A Shaolin practitioner should be able to be "Calm in defending and fierce in attacking." This concept can be found in the manual "Shaolin Boxing" written during the dynastic period in the Shaolin Temple. This book was composed by the well known martial arts masters of China through the invitation of Shaolin monks and established the foundation for *Wu*.

While at one time, hands and feet were the only expected tools of *Wu*. The many martial arts styles would later learn how to extend their natural abilities by incorporating weapons. The development of certain weapon forms were due to the incorporation of *Chan* and *Wu* into objects. Different weapons came into use such as the conventional spear and staff or the more unconventional pitchfork and chain whip. Many of these weapons were the advancement of discipline, understanding, and application of *Chan* and *Wu*.

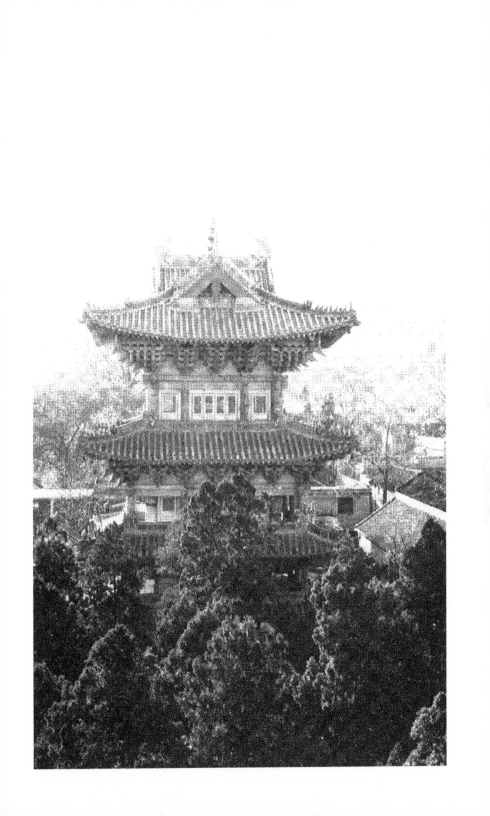

Mind and Body

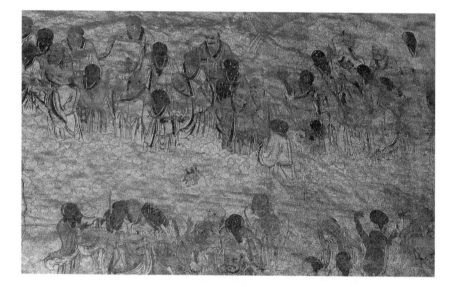

The key to understanding martial arts is to establish a strong connection between the mind and body. A balance must be maintained between both. If one falters behind the other, then both will not be able to function effectively as a single entity. A consciousness in developing the mind and body should be ideal throughout the journey through martial arts and life itself.

The body is trained through the discipline of performing the movements contained within this book. The mind is trained through an open-minded approach towards the forms. But the most important training is to become familiar with the possibilities. The goal is to enrich the soul by exposing it to the different aspects of life. When both are combined, we become more tolerant and understanding towards the unexplainable occurrences of everyday living. Many people travel from all over the world to the Shaolin Temple to seek enlightenment from the monks that live there. Yet, these monks reflect a simple way of life. They believe in devoting themselves to their actions and not the result. Through such discipline they are able to perform magnificent feats and demonstrate an invincible will power. The Shaolin monks have trained their mind and body to martial arts every day. Now ask yourself this question. Where did martial arts come from? The art has been passed down through many generations and they have spread throughout the world. This is why there is a large amount of styles and forms. In the beginning there was a necessity; the necessity of self defense and health.

The Shaolin Five Animals form was created through the observation of nature itself. The animals in their natural elements were seen performing different movements in attacking and defending. These movements were then used to create each form. Through the practice of each form, the mind captures the spirit and the body captures the strength of the particular animal. For example, a person practicing the Snake form can master the mechanics of the snake form, but the mind must capture the spirit of the snake. The mind must understand what makes a snake a snake.

As much as science and medicine have advanced, the mind and body is still a mystery, yet it has a tendency to recall memories or the familiar. Through repetition, the part of the brain that controls particular muscle movements becomes reinforced. As a result the mind and body become accustomed with the action. The five forms in this book cannot be explained in depth and in detail. Yet, through the constant repetition of the forms the individual will discover the purpose of particular chains of movements and the human body learns to become more effective with the movement and action.

With every force there is a counter force. There is a continuum between two sides that work together and separates itself from each other. The understanding of the mind and body is the understanding of cause and effect, action and reaction.

Another point of view is that the mind is formlessness and the body brings form. Martial arts has the word art in it. Art is created the same way. It is created from the abstract and given form by the hands of the artist. Music is another example. It is created by a composer that controls his or her craft in order for the music to be played.

Natural State

All humans are born naturally good. However, this state is affected by the real world. The temptation of the real world twist and cloud the individual's judgements of what is right and wrong. The moral side of a person is many things. These such things are not talking behind other's back, upholding a certain manner in public, showing respect towards each and every person, and many more. The mind and heart will always be inside us all. It is that selfishness, anger, fear, hate, and greed that cloud both. However, the heart and mind are still with us. We must attempt to find our own through the waste that we accumulate when we enter this world. The sun and the moon are always in the sky. In the beginning they are clear and visible. But when, storm clouds and dark skies cover up both it remains hard to see. It is when the clouds are scattered that the sun and moon are visible again.

Goodness is always there within us all. It is through temptation and accumulation of waste that we do not see our goodness. If one seeks to sort out one's own thoughts and life they will be able to find their true mind and heart. The realization of this respect towards oneself and others is important to the understanding of self.

The Shaolin Heart

What is it about a person's heart? Do you have the heart to do something? Are you able to push yourself? Everything in this world is a series of levels. There are so many of those that are at the lower level, but only a handful can obtain the higher levels. The first thing one must realize is that everything changes. There is no constant around you in the world. Every minute things can and will change and grow. The key is making the heart into a malleable and changeable element. One must also aim for the right and positive direction. A teacher can only train a student in a skill and teach theories and philosophies. The students bring their own attitude and discipline. This book is for all students and teaches them as equals. The ideals of the element of heart apply not only to one particular student or teacher, but to all students as a whole functioning as one. It is when students and teachers obtain this unity that martial arts flourishes.

The Basics

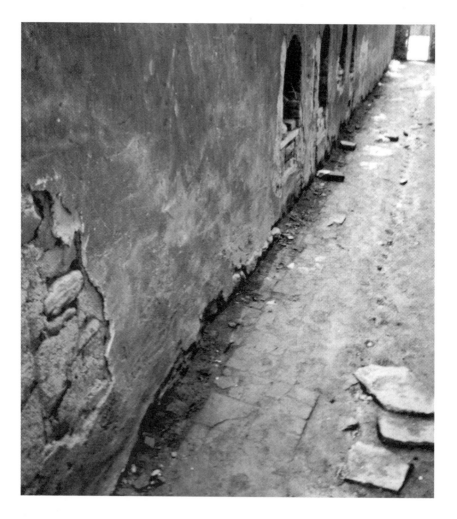

These basic exercises provide a full body work out as well as a way to develop flexibility, accuracy, and endurance. Many other aspects will follow with perseverance such as speed, agility, and strength. Basics can be compared to as the tools of the martial artist such as the types of blocks, punches and kicks. In every style of martial arts there is a core basics that ties everything else together. In every technique, form, and exercise one can be sure to notice these basics. Becoming comfortable and an expert in the basics is the key to finding the true meaning of everything discussed. It will make the difference between a person who practices martial arts to a person who is a martial artist. There is a world of difference that you will understand from experience. Every serious instructor of any martial arts style stresses the importance of the basics.

Four-Count Stretch

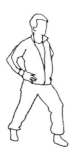 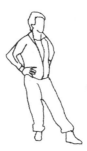

1.

Begin in a bow-and-arrow stance.

2.

Shift the weight of your body towards the back leg into a cat stance.

3.

Bend from the waist till head is close to the knee.

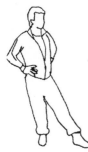 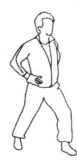

4.

Return to upright position into a cat stance.

5.

Return to a bow-and-arrow stance.

Two-Count Stretch

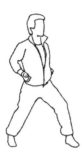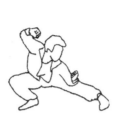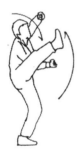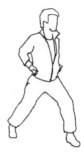

1.

Begin in a bow-and-arrow stance.

2.

Shift weight to the back leg and block.

3.

Return to a bow-and-arrow stance.

Front Leg Stretch

1.

Excute a front kick with your right leg and block high with the left hand as the right hand strikes downwards.

2.

Return to the starting position and repeat with the left leg and right hand alternating.

Nine Count Fingertip Pushup

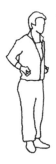

1.

Stand with feet together and back straight.

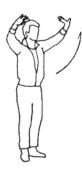

2.

Raise both hands up as high as possible.

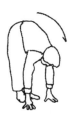

3.

Bend until both hands reach the floor.

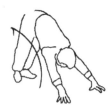

7.

Kick back into a pushup position with back straight and arms 90 degrees to your body.

8.

Make transition into a cat stretch with heels on the floor.

9.

Dive into a lowered pushup position.

4.

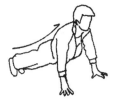

Push up from lowered position.

5.

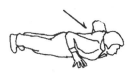

Rock back onto heels into a cat stretch with heels on the floor.

6.

At an angle stretch back into push up position. Jump with both legs unbent into position 3.

10.

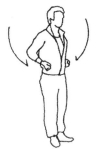

Stand up and bring both arms back to the side of your body.

Side Leg Stretch

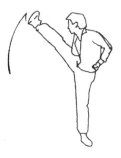 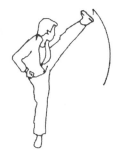

1.

Stand straight with hands on your waist, raising your right leg to the right side as high as possible.

2.

Repeat the movement using the opposite leg and alternate.

Horse Stance in Meditation

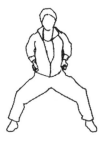 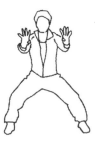 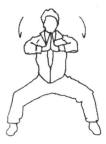

1.

Begin in a horse stance with back straight and feet parallel to each other.

2.

Extend hands out in front and fingers spread apart as far as possible. Arms bent slightly, elbows pointing down.

3.

After holding this position bring both hands together into meditation.

Straight Punch

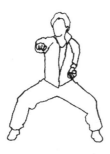 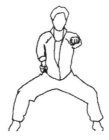

1.

Beginning in a horse stance execute a basic straight punch. Do not lock elbows.

2.

Switch to the other arm and alternate several times.

Hook Punch

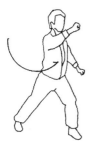 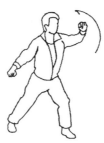 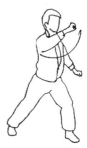

1.

Begin in a bow-and-arrow stance. Swing a hook punch with one hand and block with the opposite.

2.

Now alternate the position into another hook punch aiming towards the temple of the head.

3.

Alternate with each hand keeping in mind the attack and the block.

Uppercut

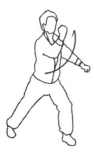 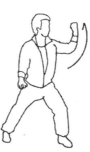 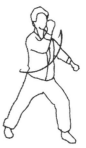

1.

Begin in a bow-and-arrow stance and block using one hand and perform a quick uppercut punch.

2.

Alternate left and right keeping track which arm is attacking and which is blocking.

3.

Repeat for several times.

Chop and Block

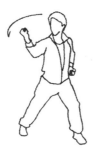 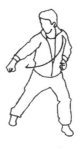

1.

From a bow-and-arrow stance using one arm, chop high from behind the ear.

2.

With the same hand, block low. From the other shoulder alternate using both arms, setting a good rhythm.

Swinging Punch

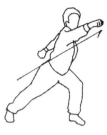

1.

Begin in a bow-and-arrow stance and a swinging punch swinging both fists upwards .

2.

Turn at the waist and rotate to the other side again moving upward with both fists.

Two Count Elbow Strike

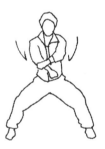

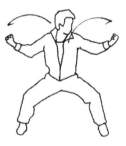

1.

In horse stance, cross both arms in front as far as possible.

2.

Bring both fists upward and strike to the sides while coming down.

Four-Count Elbow Strike

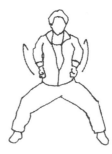

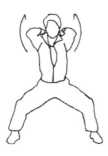

1.

In horse stance, strike upward with two forward elbow strikes.

2.

Elbows should be brought downward executing two back elbow strikes.

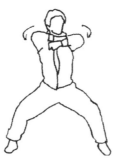

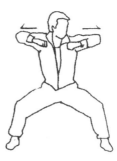

3.

Raise both arms up to form forward inward elbow strikes.

4.

With both elbows, strike to the side at the same time.

Knuckle Push-ups

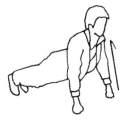

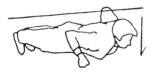

1.

Start in push-up position, the first two knuckles of each fist on the floor. Back should be straight and head should be forward.

2.

Lower the body, bend both arms until they form 90 degree angle.

Stretching

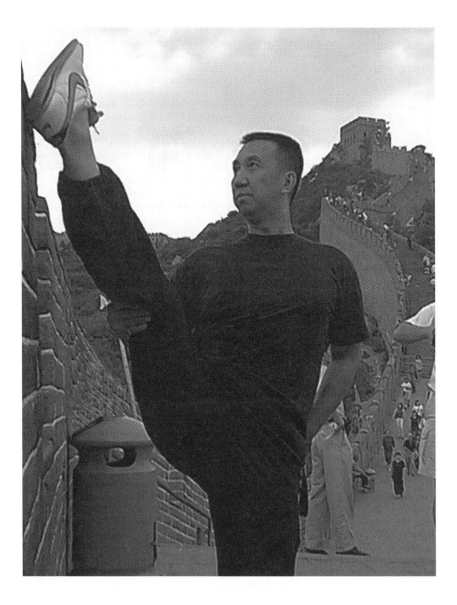

Stretching is also a factor for training. Martial arts is a very physical endeavor which one must be fully limber and flexible. Like many other physical activities, stretching avoids the cramping and spraining of muscles. Muscles are composed of fibers that tug a pull in order to execute an action. These fibers tend to be tight without the proper stretching. You muscles are not warmed up and are therefore cold. In order to warm them up these fibers must be stretched for certain amounts of time to prepare it for training. Many people devote a large amount of time to stretching. One also acquires looseness throughout time making their movements rhythmic with fluidity. Stretches should be performed before and after your training. This will aid in creating a more flexible person and avoid muscle tears as well.

Upper Body Stretch

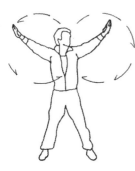 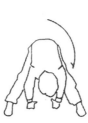 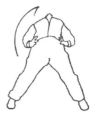

1.

Standing shoulder width apart, extend arms to the side and rotate both forward and then backwards.

2.

Bend at the waist and bring both hands to the front to touch the floor.

3.

Bring your body upright and then slowly bend back with hands on waist.

Head-to-Knee Stretch

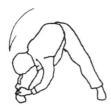 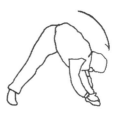

1.

Standing shoulder width apart, bring both hands toward one foot without bending knees.

2.

Do the same with the opposite foot. Repeat.

Middle Leg Stretch

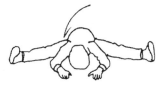 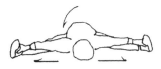

1.

Legs spread open on the floor, lean forward slowly.

2.

While in this position extend both arms to touch the toes.

Side Leg Stretch

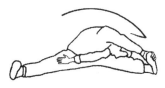

1.

Legs spread open on the floor lean to one side reaching for your toes.

2.

Do the same with the other leg. Repeat.

Extended Leg and Butterfly Stretch

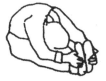 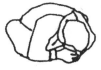

1.

With legs extend in front, bend the body over reaching with hands to touch the feet.

2.

Bring both feet in together and bend forward to slowly stretch.

Figure Four Stretch

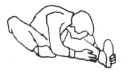 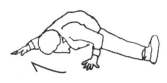

1.

Have one leg tucked inside and the other leg forward. Bend and touch both hands to foot.

2.

In same position stretch the upper body towards the opposite direction.

Stances

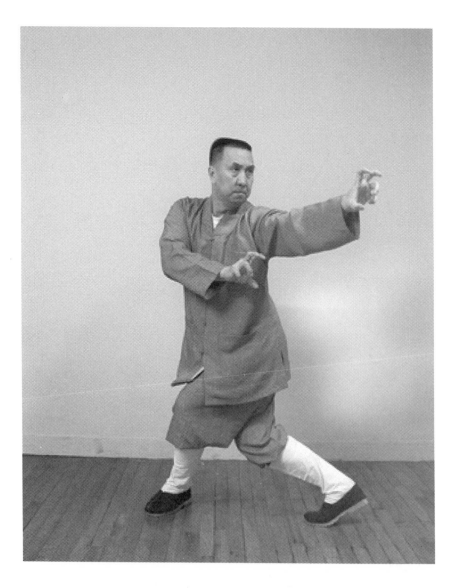

Learning the stances is the first and most basic principle of martial arts. Stances can be compared to as the roots or the foundation of martial arts. Without strong roots a tree will never grow. A house must have a strong foundation in order to stand the tests of time. To measure the success of a martial artist one can observe the performance of their stances. Without proper stances the execution of forms and techniques will not be effective and will become broken down to the point which they are showing movements with lack of meaning.

The proper executions of stances will provide stability, balance, and strength for your lower body. The details of stances and upper body movements help to align the body to change from one particular stance to another which also provides the speed and strength of your strikes from your body to the target. The center of gravity shifts and the momentum of your own body is used with your own strength to create fluid and powerful movements.

In techniques and forms which require executing movements and counter-movements, stances prove to be important in reacting to advances and retreats. The proper execution of stances will allow the person to step jump, attack, and defend in perfect balance. gain, the key to everything is balance internally and externally.

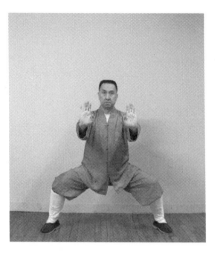

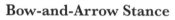

Horse Stance

1.

Stand with both legs distributing weight equally. Sit in the stance and have your back straight. Both feet should face forward and be parallel to each other.

Bow-and-Arrow Stance

2.

One leg is bent at a 90 degree angle while the other leg should be straight. The weight should be mainly on the bent leg.

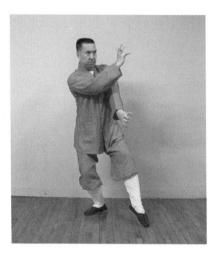

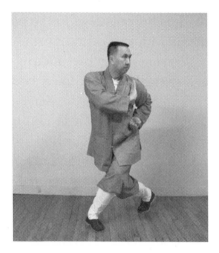

Cat Stance

4.

The weight of your body should be on the back leg and the front leg should be light as possible only letting the toe touch the floor.

X Stance

5.

This stance coils the leg up for a quick retreat. Both legs should be crossed to resemble the X and the weight should be equally distributed.

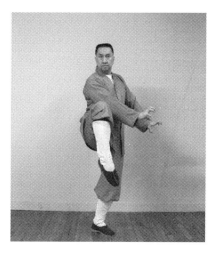

Crane Stance

3.

This stance mimics a crane standing on one leg. The weight should be on leg while the other leg should be as high as possible and bent at the knee.

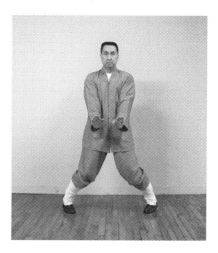

A Stance

6.

This is a transition stance moving from one stance to another. Both knees should face inward and towards each other.

The Five Animals

Dragon Form

The dragon is the first animal of the Shaolin five animal forms. Although existence of dragons are only legends, it has long been believed to symbolize grace and beauty along with tremendous power. In Chinese mythology, the dragon comes from water and its movements are very fluid and circular. The dragon style uses its claws to grab and hold while delivering a powerful blow with another part of the body, or using its body to produce a leverage against opponents. Much of the power comes from the circular twisting movement of the body. Such movement is also influenced by the development of the internal powers of the body.

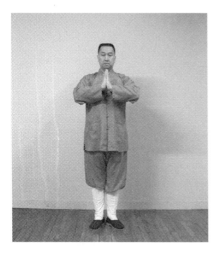

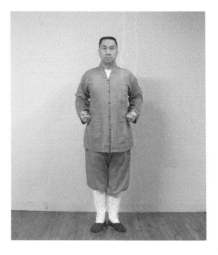

1. Feet are together, back is straight, and both hands in meditation.

2. Hands to the side from meditation.

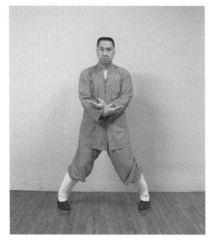

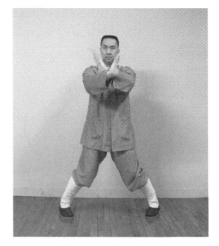

5. Arms in an X block. Legs in A stance close together.

6. A high X block with both hands.

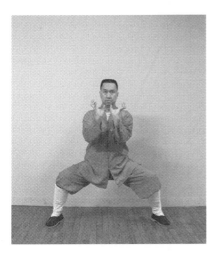

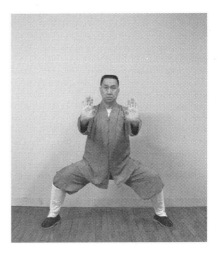

3. Legs in horse stance, dragon claws to block in front.

4. Double palm strike to the front.

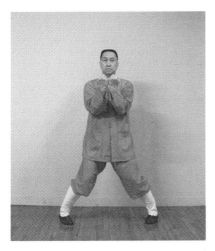

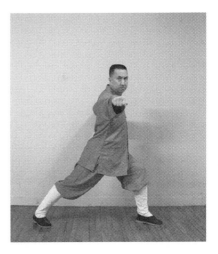

7. Block high with both arms.

8. Bow-and-arrow stance, double side punches.

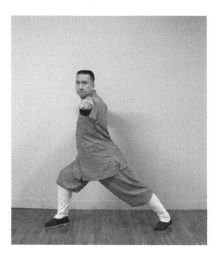

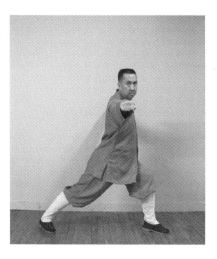

9. Bow-and-arrow stance to the opposite direction, double side punch again.

10. Repeat position 8 again in a bow-and arrow-stance.

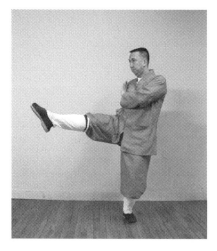

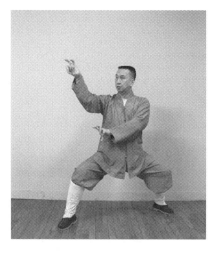

13 Front kick with the right leg to waist level.

14. Double dragon claws in a horse stance.

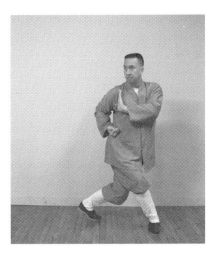

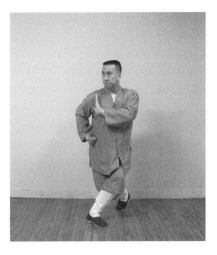

11. X stance and side block with left palm.

12. Hands in place, step over with left leg into X stance.

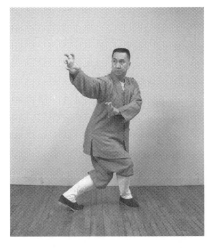

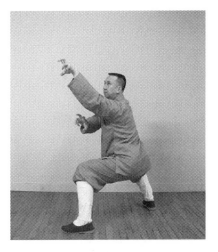

15. Hands in same position, step back into X stance.

16. Step into horse stance with double dragon claws.

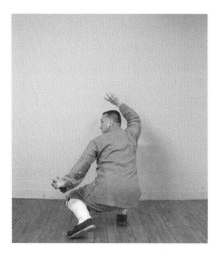 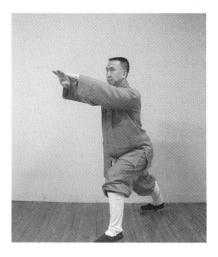

17. Underhand claw strike and block and retreat into a crouching stance.

18. Bow and arrow stance, both arms in front with hands together.

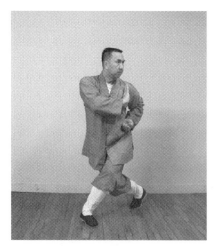 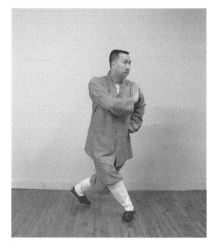

21. Step into X stance with the left leg and a side palm block.

22. Cross into X stance with right leg, arms in same position.

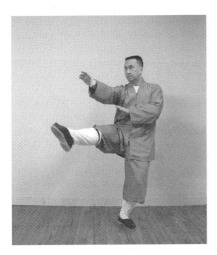

19. Right front kick to waist level Touch foot with right hand.

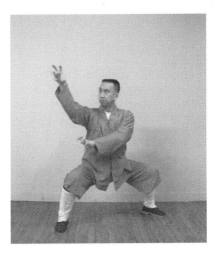

20 Horse stance and double dragon claws.

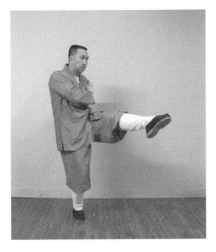

23. Front kick to waist level and palm block.

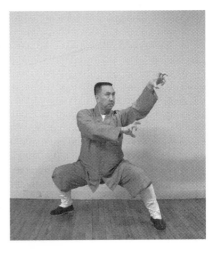

24. Horse stance and double dragon claw.

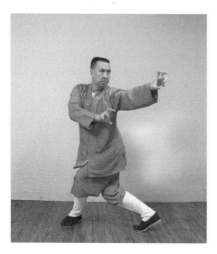

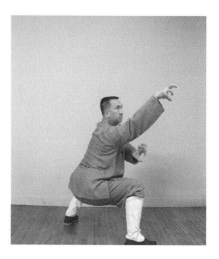

25. Left leg crosses into X stance, both hands still in double dragon claws.

26. Pivot and rotate into horse stance.

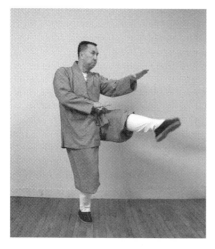

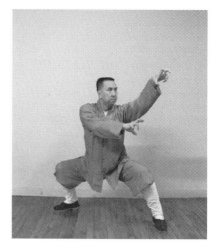

29. Left front kick to the waist, left hand should touch foot.

30. Step into horse stance with double dragon claws.

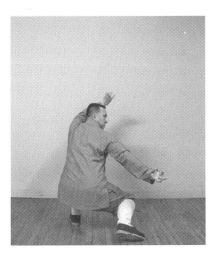

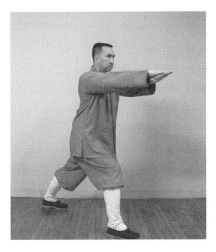

27. Retreat into crouching stance with underhand dragon claw and block to the head.

28. Arms forward and hands together into a bow and arrow stance.

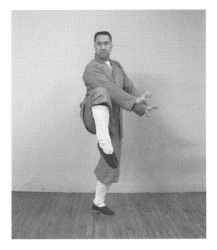

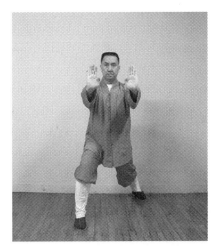

31. Right leg crane stance with double hand grab to the side.

32. Double palm strike in bow and arrow stance.

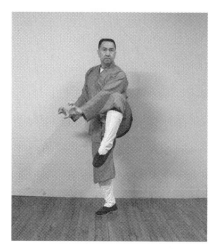

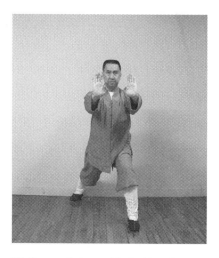

33. Left leg crane stance with double hand grab to the side.

34. Bow and arrow with double palm strike.

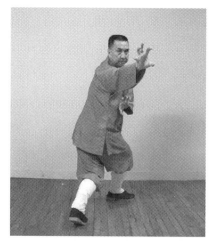

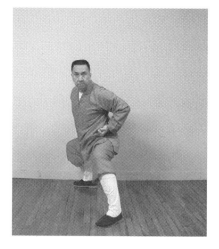

37. Retreat in X stance and defensive block.

38. Turn right into a horse stance and hands to the side of the body.

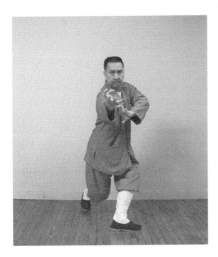

35. Twist into X stance with double dragon claw grab.

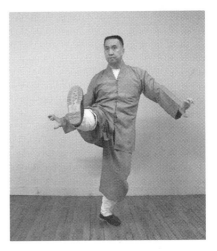

36. Front kick with two hand grab.

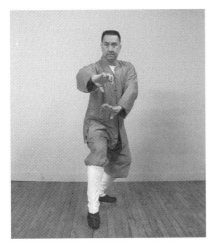

39. Cat stance with double hand grab.

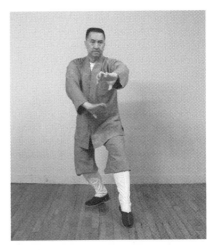

40. Step back with right foot into cat stance with double hand grab.

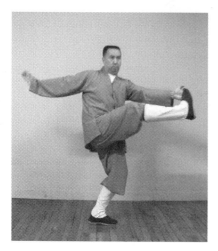

41. Crescent kick with right leg.

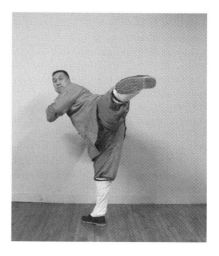

42. Momentum should carry you into a side kick.

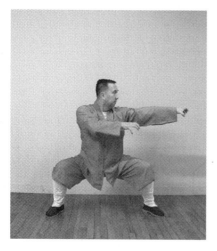

45. Horse stance and double raking claws to the left.

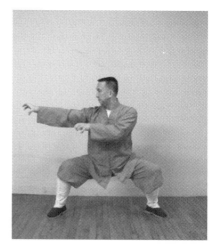

46. Horse stance and double raking claws to the right now.

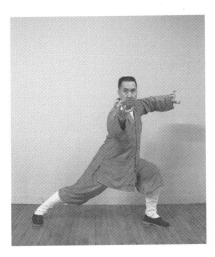

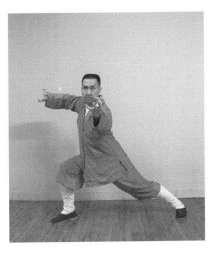

43. Horse stance with underhand dragon claw.

44. Repeat again in the opposite direction.

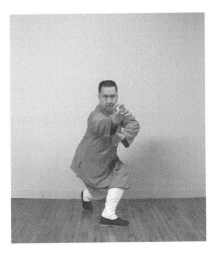

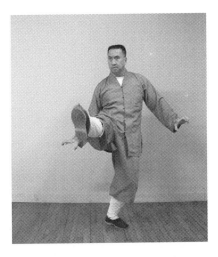

47. Move to X stance with double grappling claws.

48. Front kick with double arm grab.

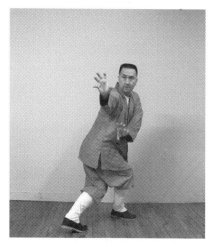 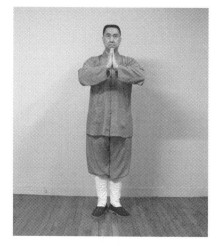

49. Retreating X stance with double dragon claw block.

50. End the form in the opening stance with hands back in meditation.

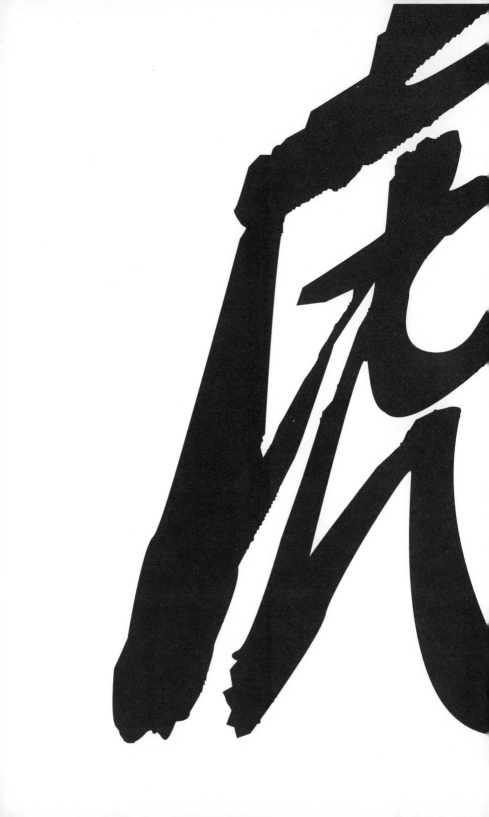

Tiger Form

The tiger is the second animal in the five animal set and one of the most powerful. The tiger is an animal that is known for its speed, agility and external strength. Training under this form will develop the bones, joints, and tendons as it requires intricate coordinated movements. The body is trained in the manner where it holds in twisting stances to develop a coil like exertion. This centers the body to the ground and develops the legs to become more graceful yet deadly. This form is perhaps the most physically challenging of all the forms. Mastery of this form will strengthen the forearms, legs, torso and hands.

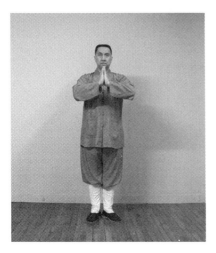

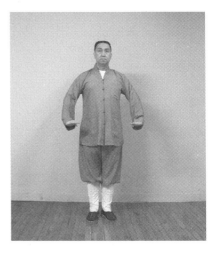

1. Begin in a meditation stance and feet together.

2. Both arms to the side with palms facing down.

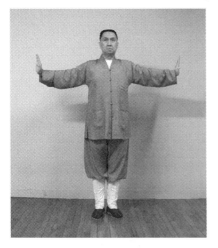

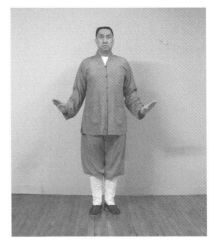

5. Using dynamic tension bring both hands out straight to the side.

6. Bring arms down and tuck them to the side.

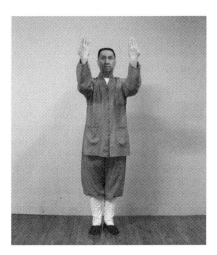

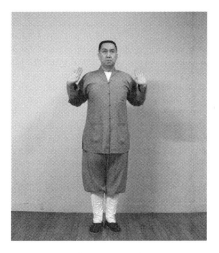

3. Double front hand block. Both palms are facing you.

4. Both arms tucked and hands close to shoulders.

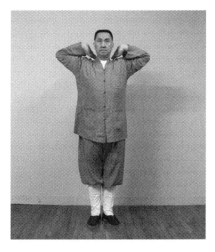

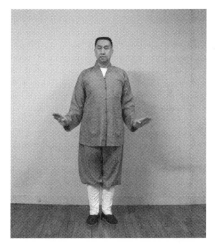

7. Double high elbow strike with hands tucked in.

8. Sunken hands with arms tucked to the sides.

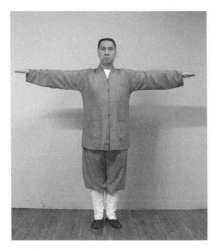

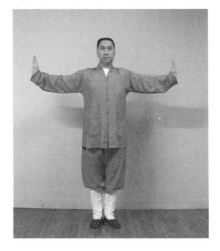

9. Double spear hands to the side of the body.

10. Bring both hands up and palms facing the side.

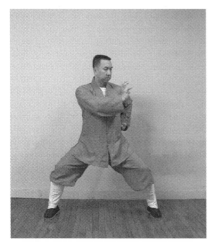

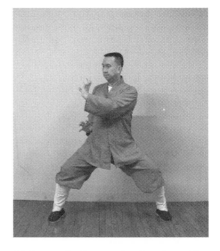

13. Open into horse stance and right tiger claw in front of you.

14. Repeat in the opposite direction with the other hand.

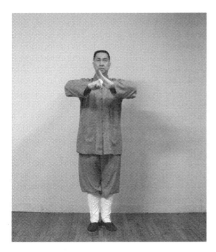

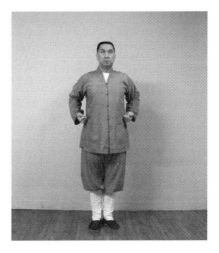

11. Both hands in open bowing stance to show respect.

12. Return both hands to the side of the body or in chamber. Back is straight.

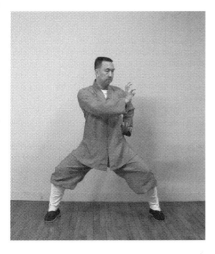

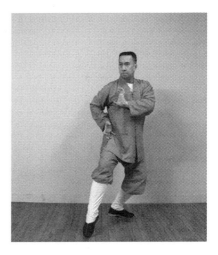

15. Repeat again with the right hand in tiger claw.

16. Retreat with cat stance and double tiger claw block.

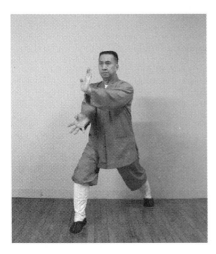

17. Forward with bow and arrow stance and double butterfly palm.

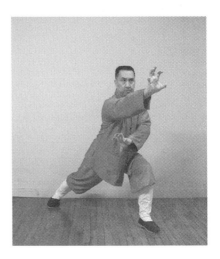

18. Switch left bow and arrow stance. Attack with double tiger claws with right hand leading.

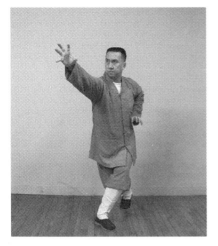

21. Step forward with left leg into X stance and right leading tiger claw.

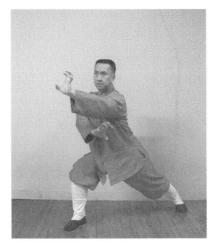

22. Bow and arrow stance with a tiger claw block and strike.

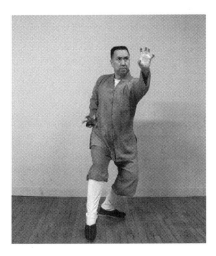

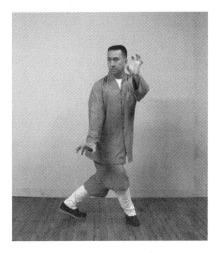

19. Step up into a cat stance and left tiger claw.

20. Cross step with right leg into an X stance and a tiger claw block and grab.

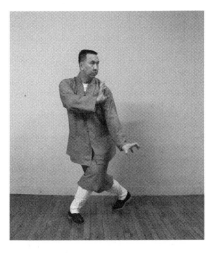

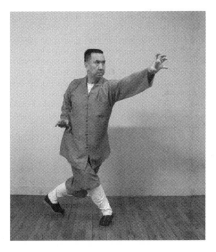

23. Retreat with an X stance and tiger claw block.

24. Step over with right leg into X stance with a left tiger claw leading.

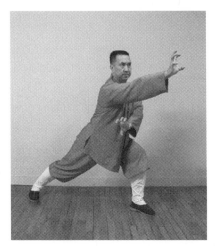

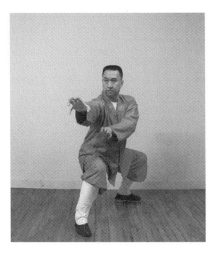

25. Advance into a bow and arrow stance with a block and strike with tiger claw.

26. Sit into a horse stance and a double hand grab.

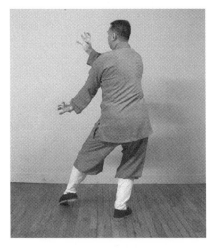

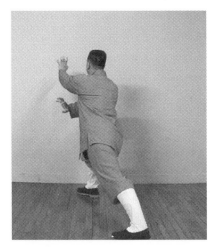

29. Cat stance into an adjusted underhand tiger claw and strike.

30. Advance into bow and arrow stance with a tiger claw block and strike.

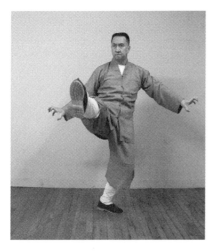

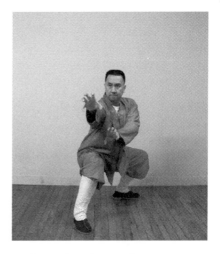

27. Pull hands apart and perform a front kick.

28. Retreat into the same horse stance position and tiger claw grab.

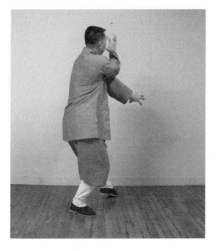

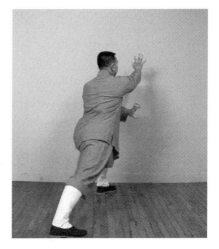

31. Reverse cat stance with double cross ing tiger claw attack.

32. Advance into bow and arrow and block and strike tiger claw.

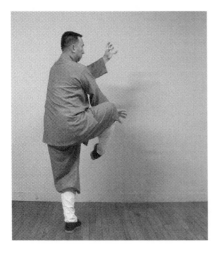

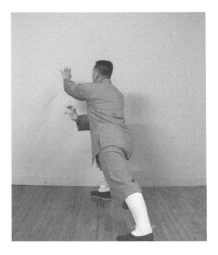

33. Retreat into a crane stance and double locking tiger claw.

34. Forward bow and arrow with block and strike with tiger claw. Left hand is leading.

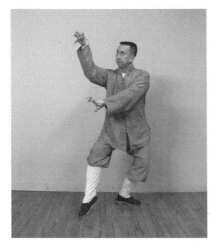

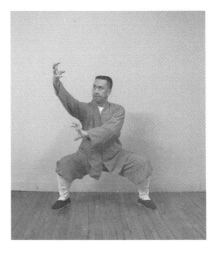

37. Retreat into a cat stance and double tiger claw grab.

38. Horse stance with double tiger claw block and hook.

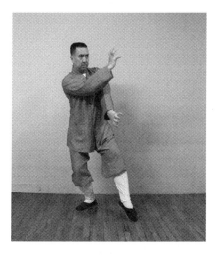

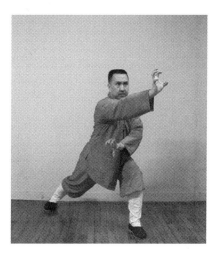

35. Pivot in cat stance with double crossing tiger claws.

36. Bow and arrow with tiger claw grab and strike.

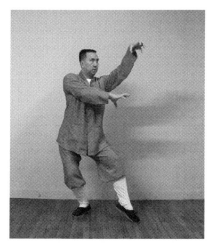

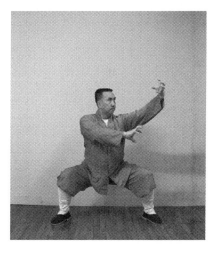

39. Cat stance with double grappling tiger claws.

40. Sit in horse stance with double tiger claw.

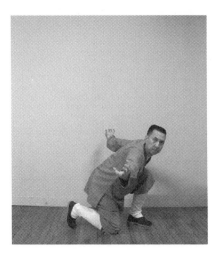

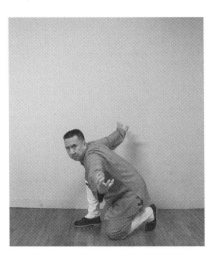

41. Crouching stance with spreading tiger claws to the side.

42. Repeat switching to the opposite side.

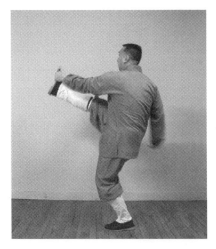

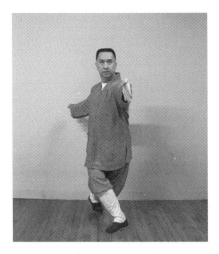

45. Pivot into a back crescent hook kick, use the left hand to hit the right foot.

46. In X stance and double open palms.

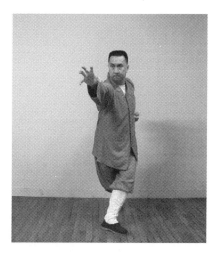

43. Retreating tiger claw strike in X stance.

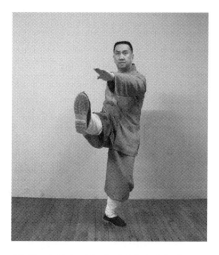

44. Front kick with the left hand. Left hand should touch the foot.

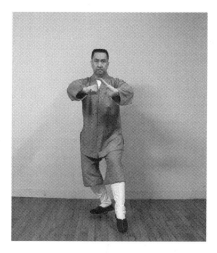

47. Step back into the same opening bow.

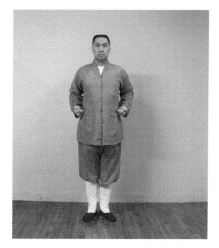

48. Return to the beginning position with hands tucked to the side.

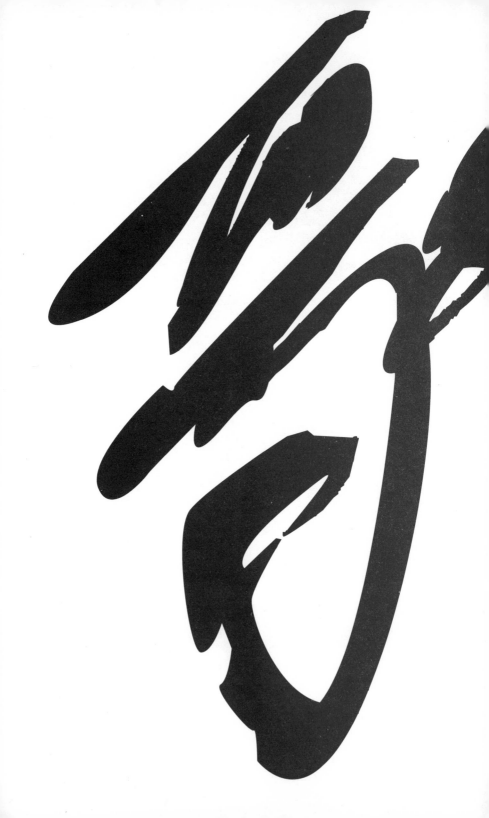

Leopard Form

The leopard form is the third animal of the five animal forms of Shaolin. It does not emphasize as much power as the tiger form, the leopard form combines speed and agile footwork to outmaneuver its opponents. It also uses a coordinated combination of short and quick strikes to confuse its opponent. The leopard moves ever so slightly to evade and deflect an opponents attack and pinpoints an opening. The footwork for this form will develop a greater balance and reaction time.

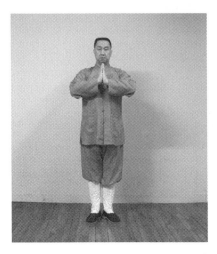

1. Begin in a meditative stance with hands and feet together.

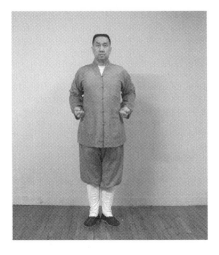

2. Bring hands to chamber to the side of your body.

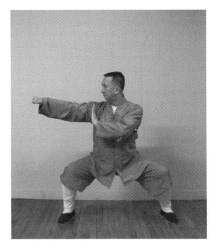

5. Horse stance with block to the chest and side punch.

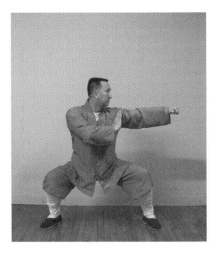

6. Repeat in the opposite direction in a horse stance still.

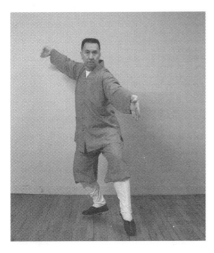

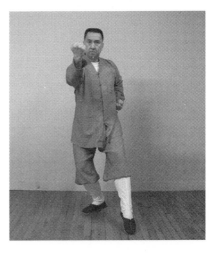

3. Begin with both hands opening to the side. Feet in cat stance.

4. Right hand performs an uppercut.

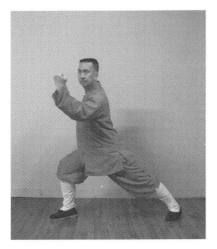

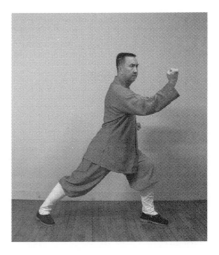

7. Bow and arrow stance with an uppercut.

8. Left bow and arrow stance with right uppercut.

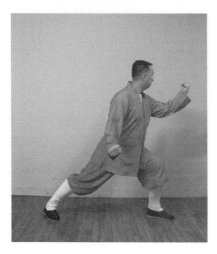

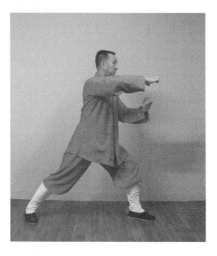

9. Left uppercut and right blocks to the side.

10. Right hand rotate around left uppercut.

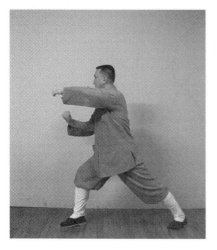

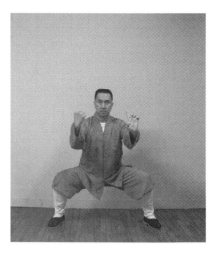

13. Left hand rotates around the right uppercut.

14. Similar dynamic tension movement and sitting in horse stance.

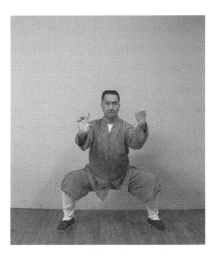

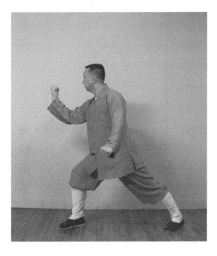

11. Dynamic tension with both hands and sitting in a horse stance.

12. Right bow and arrow stance and right uppercut while left blocks.

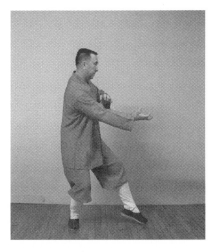

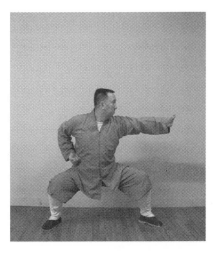

15. Cat stance with underhand leopard claw.

16. Advance into horse stance and side palm strike.

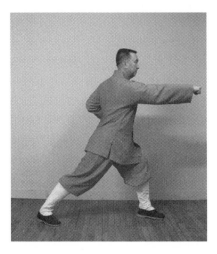

17. Forward bow and arrow and right straight punch.

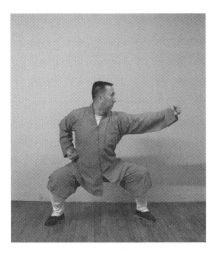

18. Horse stance with left handed sun fist.

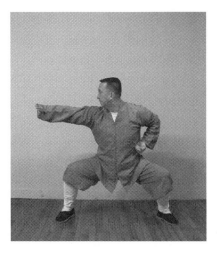

21. Horse stance with a right side palm strike.

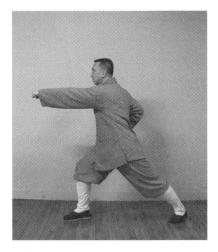

22. Left straight punch with a bow and arrow stance.

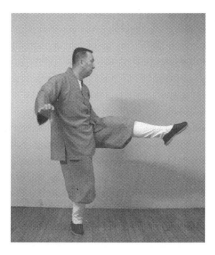

19. Open leopard claw grab and front kick.

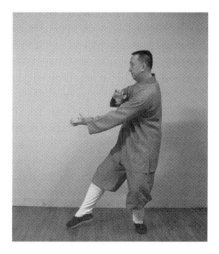

20. Left underhand leopard claw in cat stance.

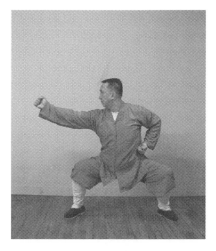

23. Right sun fist and horse stance.

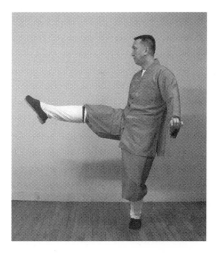

24. Double leopard claw grab and front kick.

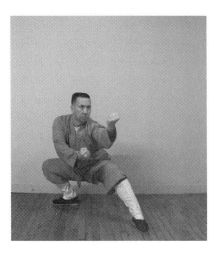

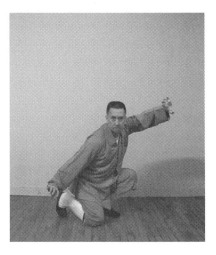

25. Low stance with double fist strike.

26. Retreat into low kneeling stance with double spread Leopard claw.

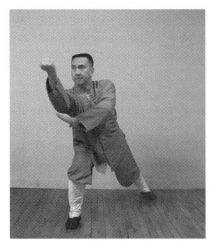

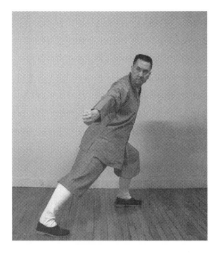

29. Spring into bow and arrow stance with underhand right punch.

30. Underhand grab and bow and arrow stance to the left.

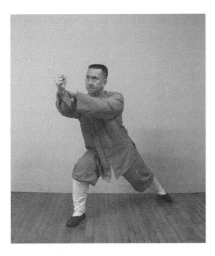

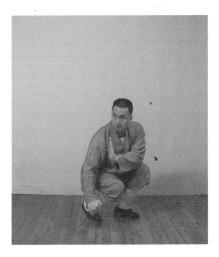

27. Forward bow and arrow stance with a held right straight punch.

28. Kneeling stance with blocking fist and palm.

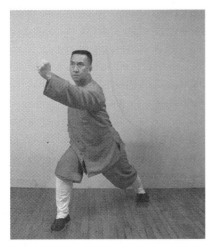

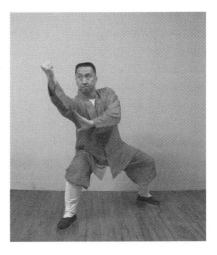

31. Forward bow and arrow and straight punch.

32. Horse stance and right straight punch.

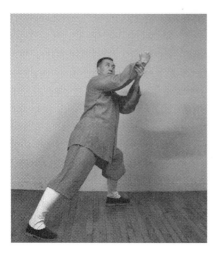

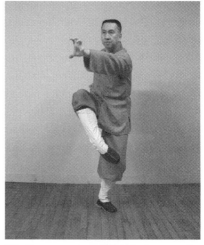

33. Retreat in a bow-and-arrow stance and fist grab.

34. Crane stance and double downward tiger claws.

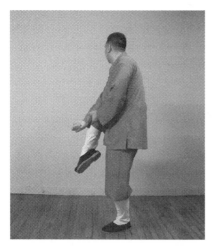

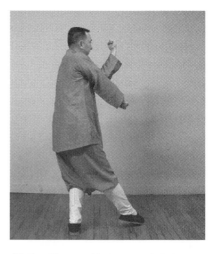

37. Crane stance and right knee block.

38. Double cross block to the right in cat stance.

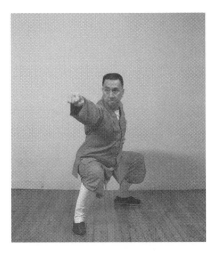

35. Horse stance and straight right punch.

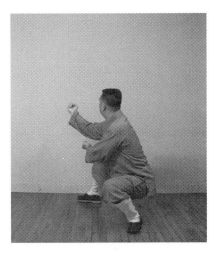

36. Turn around into low horse stance and double fist strikes.

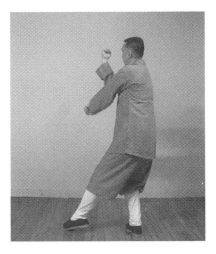

39. Double cross block and cat stance in opposite direction.

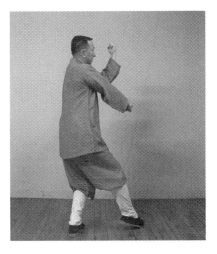

40. Repeat in opposite direction again with double hand cross block.

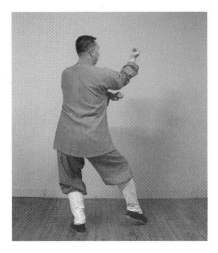

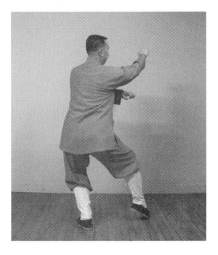

41. Double leopard claw block to the right in cat stance.

42. Cat stance with double leopard strike.

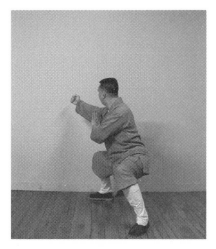

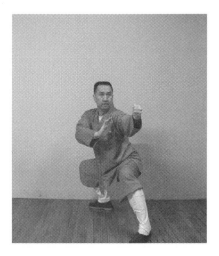

45. Horse stance and right straight punch with left palm block.

46. Turn around in horse stance and left punch and right palm block.

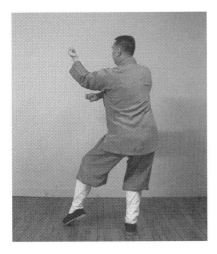

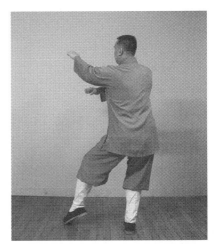

43. Double leopard claw block in opposite direction in cat stance.

44. Double leopard claw strike in cat stance.

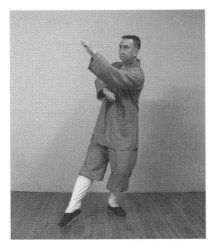

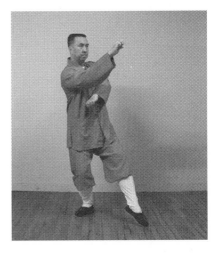

47. Left leopard claw strike and right block in cat stance.

48. Cat stance in opposite direction with right leopard claw strike and left block.

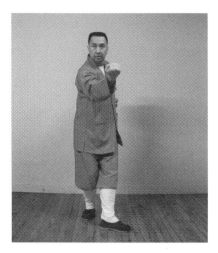

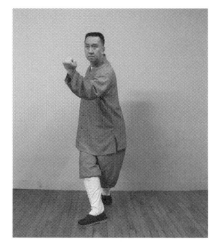

49. Right back fist in X stance. Left hand at the side.

50. Left back fist with X stance and right hand on the side.

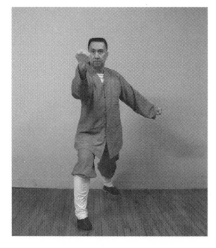

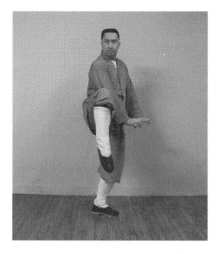

53. Right uppercut and left side block in bow-and-arrow stance.

54. Crane stance with double hand grab.

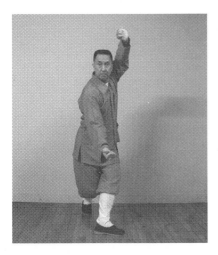

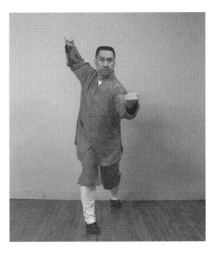

51. X stance with left head block and low right block.

52. Swinging punch in bow-and-arrow stance.

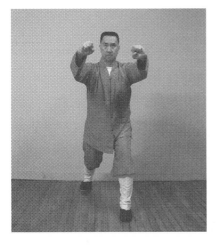

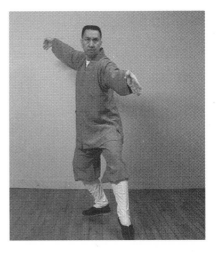

55. Left bow-and-arrow stance with double head strikes.

56. Open into a double hand block to front and back in a cat stance.

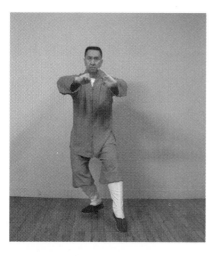 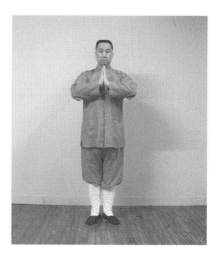

57. Finishing bow in cat stance.

58. Return to the beginning position.

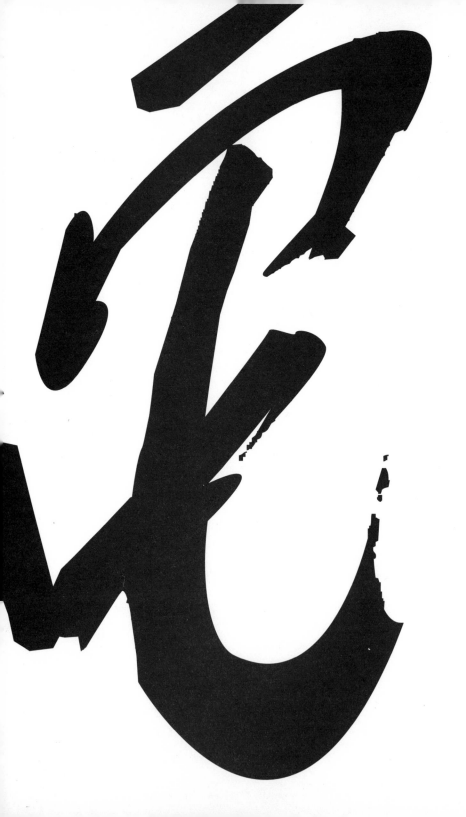

Snake Form

The snake form is very different from all the other animal forms. The snake does not have any legs or claws, which means its power comes from coiling its body and exploding to strike an opponent. The snake style uses the fingertips and palm strike to attack an opponent's pressure points. The different strikes in this form are meant to be offensive and defensive at the same time. The snake form focuses on internal energy and the release of power from the waist. This form is the opposite of the tiger form. Where as the tiger style uses hard powerful blocks and strikes. The snake uses a soft and quick approach using internal power.

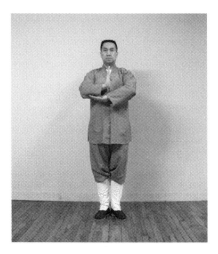

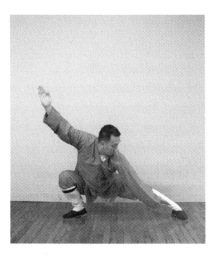

1. Opening bow with snake hands.

2. Low back stance with open snake hands to the left side.

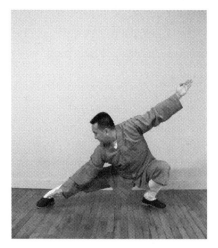

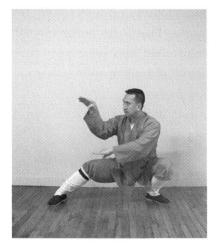

5. Repeat again to the right side.

6. Sit into a low semi-back stance with double snake hand block.

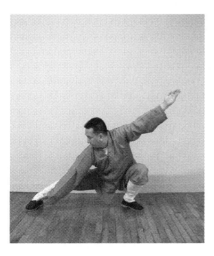

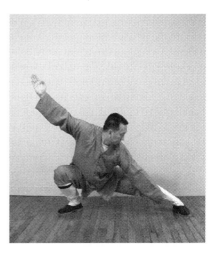

3. Low back stance and open snake hands to the right side.

4. Repeat to the left side again with open snake hands.

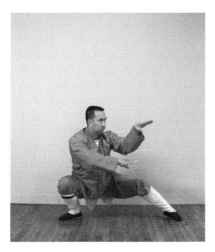

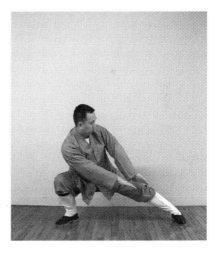

7. Shift weight to the right side with double snake hand block.

8. Low snake hand strike in back stance.

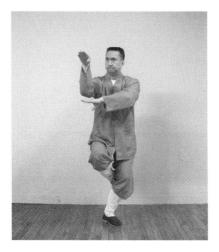

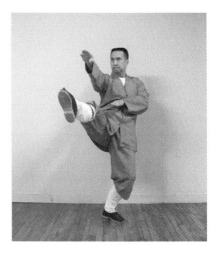

9. Right foot tucked behind the left knee with left snake hand block and right snake hand strike.

10. Right front kick and right snake hand strike.

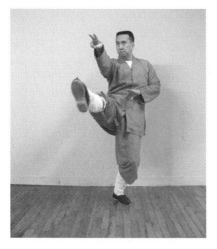

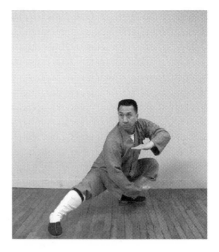

13. Front kick with right hand snake eyes strike.

14. Retreat in low back stance and double coiled snake hands.

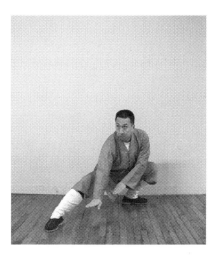

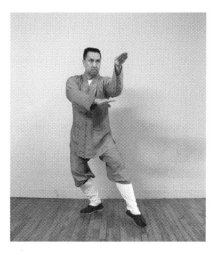

11. Low stance and double snake hand retreat.

12. Double snake hand block in cat stance.

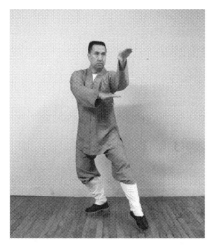

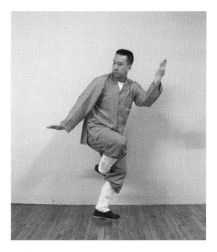

15. Double snake hand block in cat stance.

16. Retreat with right backhand snake strike.

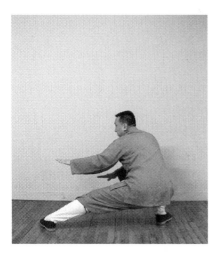

17. Turn around into low stance and low snake hands.

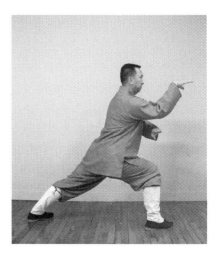

18. Rotate and stand in bow-and-arrow stance with double snake hands.

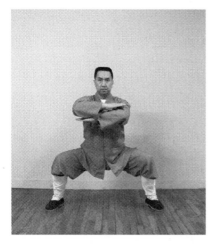

21. Turn around into horse stance with right arm on top of left.

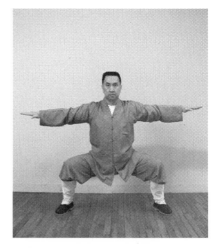

22. Spread both hands to the side in horse stance.

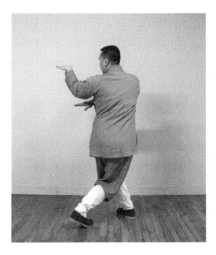

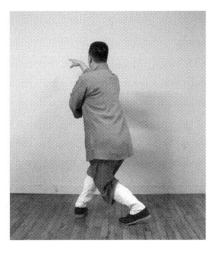

19. X stance with double snake hand block.

20. Cross into X stance and double snake hand with opposite hands.

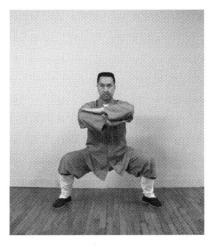

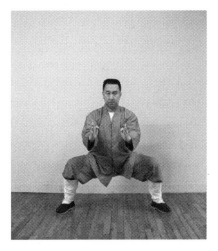

23. Left arm on top of right in horse stance.

24. Double hand chop in horse stance.

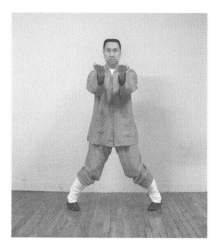

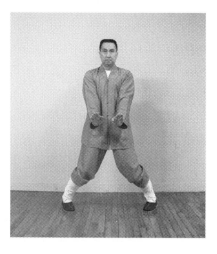

25. Raise both hands to shoulder level and stand in an A stance.

26. Double palm strike in an A stance.

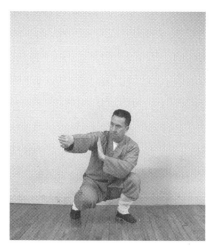

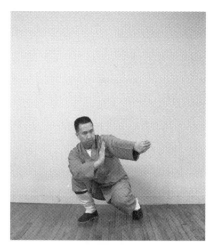

29. Low stance with low right snake hand strike.

30. Low stance with low left snake hand strike.

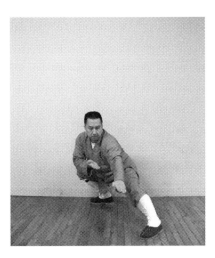

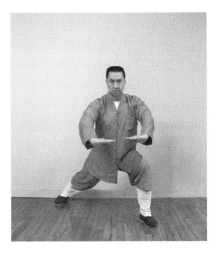

27. Double snake hand low block and low stance.

28. Double hand block with bow-and-arrow stance.

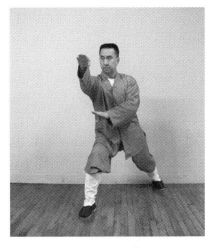

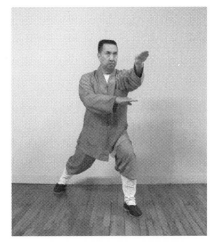

31. Upward right snake hand strike in bow-and-arrow stance.

32. Switch into left bow-and-arrow stance and left snake hand.

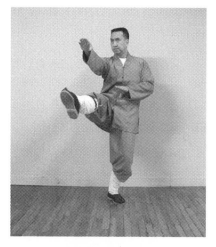

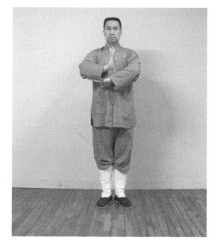

33. Front right kick and right snake hand.

34. Return to the beginning position.

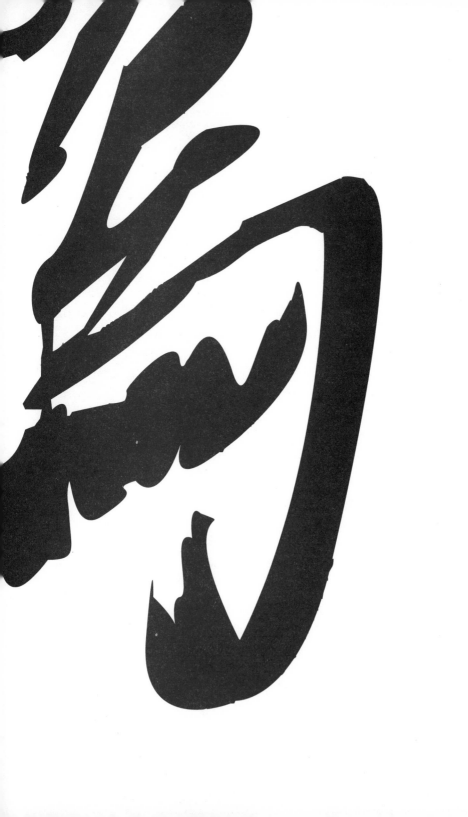

Crane Form

The crane form is the fifth form within the five animal forms. The crane itself is a patient and quick animal. It has the ability to stand on one leg for many hours and not move. This is a testament to its concentration and focus. Its ability to defeat an opponent comes from its ability to hook an attackers blow, divert them, and counter attack from close or afar. The crane hand focuses on the precision of each strike. The wide and circular swinging movements emphasize the circular motions of the wings and the legs of the crane. The crane form is effective in training the fingers, arms, and legs.

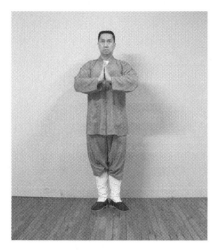

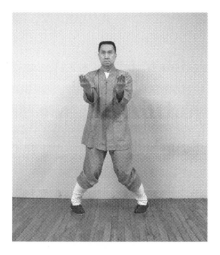

1. Beginning opening stance.

2. Open in an A stance with both palms facing up.

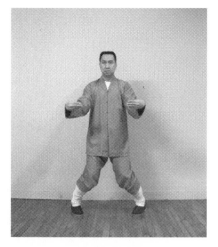

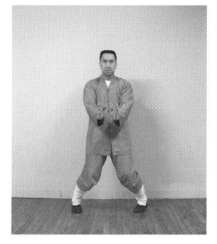

5. Double crane hand in an A stance.

6. Double palm strike in an A stance.

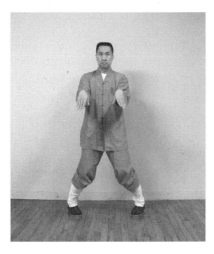

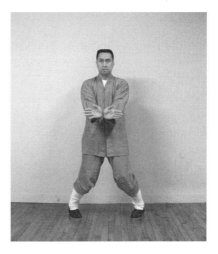

3. Bring both palms down remaining in an A stance.

4. Double palm strike in A stance.

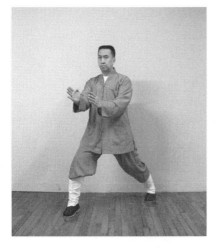

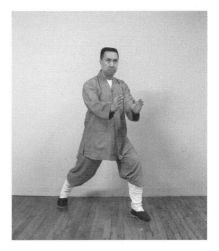

7. Bow-and-arrow stance with double spear hand.

8. Bow and arrow stance with double spear hand in opposite direction..

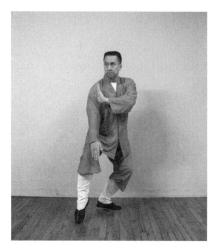

9. Retreat with low palm block.

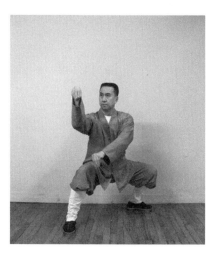

10. Attack with double crane strike in horse stance.

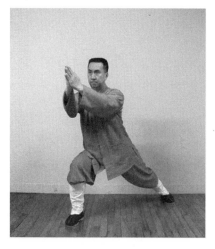

13. Double buddha strike in bow-and-arrow stance.

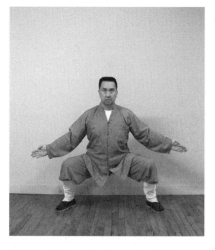

14. Sit with both hands to the side in horse stance.

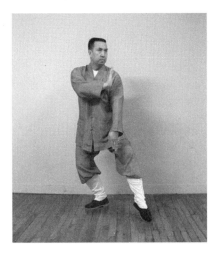

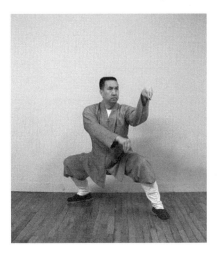

11. Retreat on opposite side with low palm block into cat stance.

12. Advance with double crane strike in horse stance.

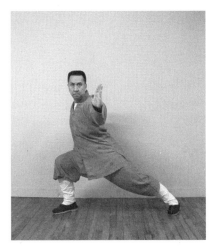

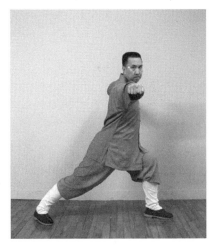

15. Left hand palm strike to the front in bow-and-arrow stance.

16. Double punch to the side in bow-and-arrow stance.

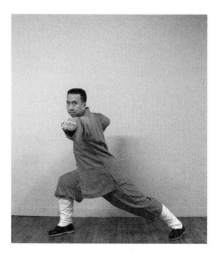

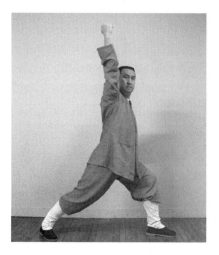

17. Repeat in opposite direction in bow-and-arrow stance.

18. Right high uppercut in bow-and-arrow stance.

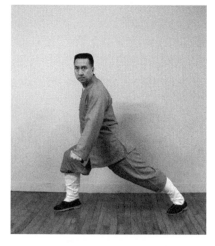

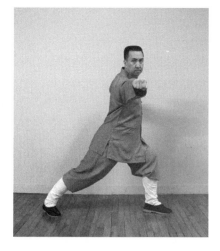

21. Left downward punch in opposite bow-and-arrow stance.

22. Double punch in bow-and-arrow stance.

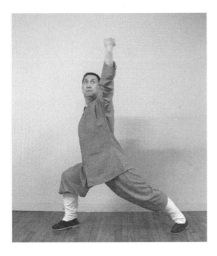

19. Repeat with left hand in bow arrow stance.

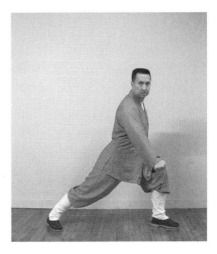

20. Downward right punch in bow-and-arrow stance.

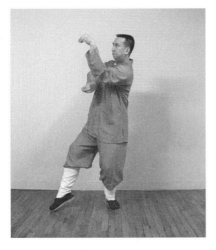

23. Double crane strike in cat stance.

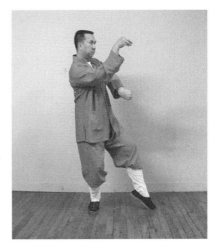

24. Double crane strike in opposite direction in cat stance.

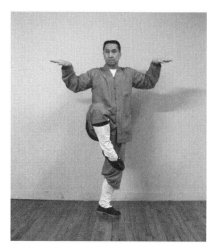

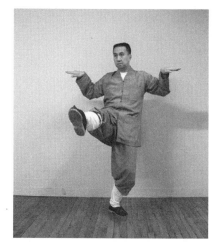

25. Open winged crane in a crane stance.

26. Front kick with double crane wings.

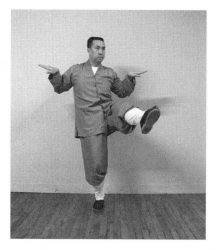

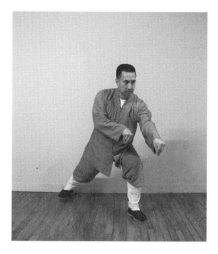

29. Front kick with crane wings.

30. Low crane strike with bow and arrow stance.

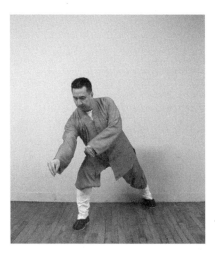

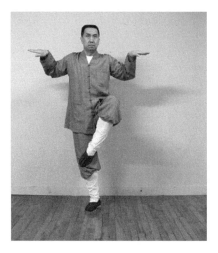

27. Bow and arrow with low right crane strike.

28. Open winged crane in crane stance with left leg.

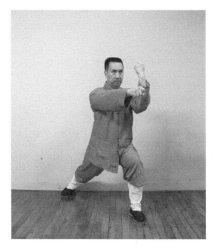

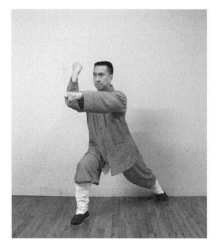

31. Block and punch in bow and arrow stance.

32. Block and punch with bow and arrow to the right.

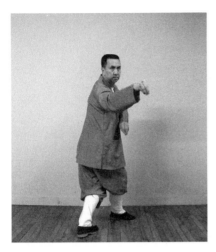

33. Retreat in an X stance and double crane block.

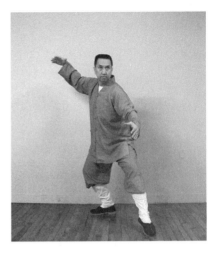

34. Both hands open in a cat stance.

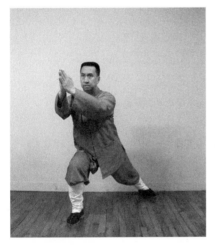

37. Double hand spear in a bow and arrow stance.

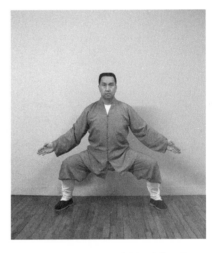

38. Sit in horse stance with both hands to the lower sides.

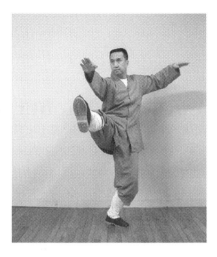

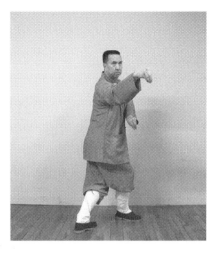

35. Double kick with right hand touching the foot.

36. Retreat in X stance with double crane block.

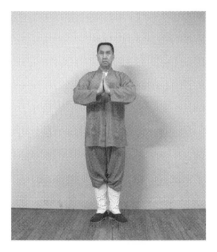

39. Return to the starting open position.

Student and Teacher

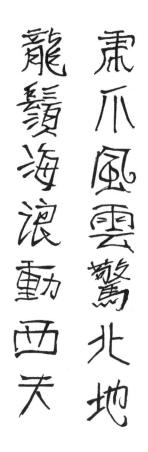

This book has provided a glimpse into the intricate workings of the Shaolin Five Animals. This journey that each student takes is full of obstacles that they must surpass. With a strong mind and a body to execute.

During the year, Russell Wong, one of Sifu Tak Wah Eng's student traveled to Tibet to meet the Dalai Lama at his temple. He tells this story to Sifu Eng about his experience and what he had seen.

The journey into the temple involved a 10-hour drive through many different locations in the countryside. The small van carried a small group of tourists that would eventually enter one of the most spiritual locations in Tibet. Getting to their location would prove more difficult than expected. There were many back roads and undefined paths through the mountainous areas.

Many people travel to meet the Dalai Lama in order to obtain his holy blessing and enlightenment. When Russell arrived at the temple he saw that a huge line formed in front of the courtyard waiting to be received. When Russell finally met him he felt a strong impression from the Dalai Lama. He described his presence as an aura of peacefulness. With this meeting Russell was able to spend time with him praying and meditating from dusk till dawn. Through this close interaction, it felt as if an energy was passed along from both individuals.

As the day passed into the late night, the Dalai Lama accompanied the guests back to the small village at the bottom of the mountainous region. Yet, without any daylight, navigating through the road became more treacherous. As time passed, everyone in the car became more uneasy as the road became more winding and bumpy. Russell could not help but feel the same way. He looked to the Dalai Lama to realize that he was unfazed by his surroundings. He maintained a calm and natural state. With such a reaction to his environments, it began to affect everyone else. Through example the Dalai Lama calmed everyone's fears through his own calmness.

As the small group reached the village they would stop for the night, they found a small inn for everyone. In his room that night, Russell had been wrestling with his own state of mind. A troubling doubt was in his heart that kept him up. With the sense of unrest he went to the Dalai Lama and entered his room. He found the Llama

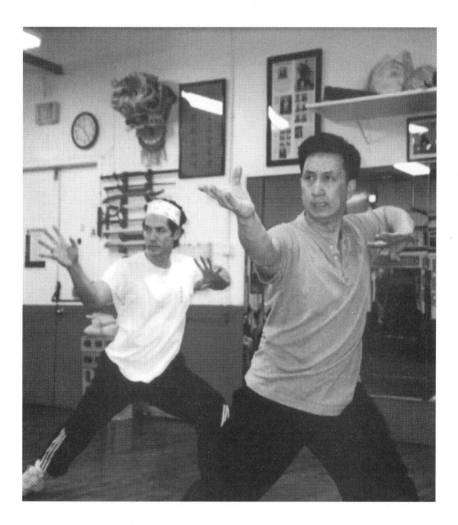

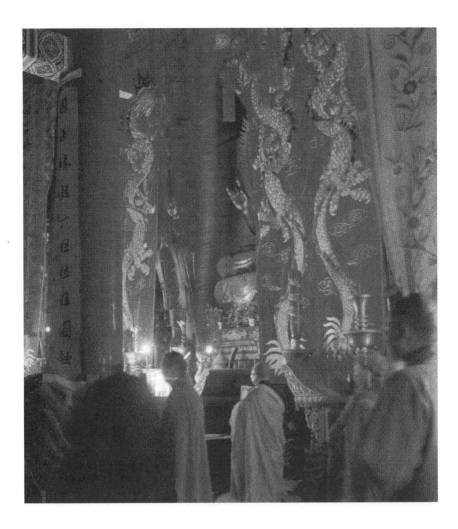

praying and in deep meditation. Russell asked for his guidance about the uneasiness in his soul. The Dalai Lama told him that he anticipated him to come to talk that night. Through some soft spoken words and a graceful hand he handed his own prayer beads to Russell. They began to meditate and chant together in order to calm both their souls. After the meditative session, the Dalai Lama told Russell that in the past he had played the role of an emperor. A chosen one that had a strong persona. He also said that Russell had a deeper and more powerful path to follow in his life. This path would lead to an enriching life within himself and the people around him.

After that night, Russell began to see things in a new perspective. The soft spoken words would always be remembered by him. Within those words a new confidence would be gained. He remembered the whole experience from the beginning to the end. His eyes were more opened to the world around him. The enlightenment he gained restored his faith in himself and the life around him. To this day Russell still carries the words of the Dalai Lama in his heart and in his mind.

As told by Russell Wong to Sifu Tak Wah Eng

It is fairly common to see the youths of this world participating in various sports, activities, and hobbies in order to gain a wider scope of knowledge within their lives or to establish a familiarity in a certain set of skills that may prove to be useful later in life. Still, others search for the plethora of experiences and friends that are found and made while participating in such activities. Whatever the purposes of one's involvement with sports and hobbies may be, it is very rare that any of these activities would prove to fulfill every single one of these possibilities. For me, Kung Fu has not only been a source of experience, expertise, skills, friends, and knowledge, but an event of my life that can only be set apart from all other extracurricular activities. To the ignorant, it may seem like an activity that likens to the physical aspects of a sport, or even the lack of commitment that might be found in a hobby. However, Kung Fu shares more characteristics with the precision and mastery of art, and yet it manages to stretch even deeper.

My initial experience with martial arts and Master Tak Wah Eng had stemmed from the fact that my father was also a student of his. Having learned a great amount of knowledge and wisdom from his experiences at the school, he wished for me to gain the same understanding and expertise that would prove to be invaluable throughout my entire life. Furthermore, he also wished to continue the martial arts through his lineage, beginning with my introduction to the school. Martial arts will become an immortal

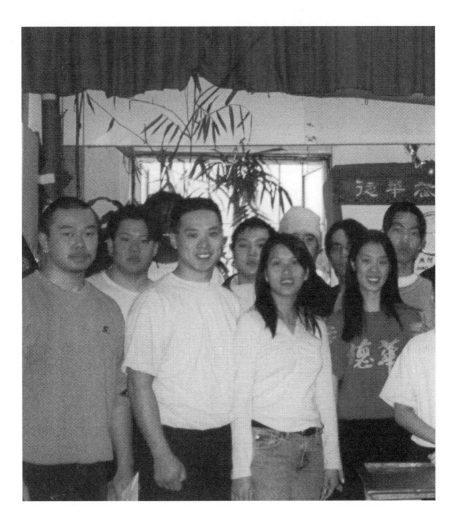

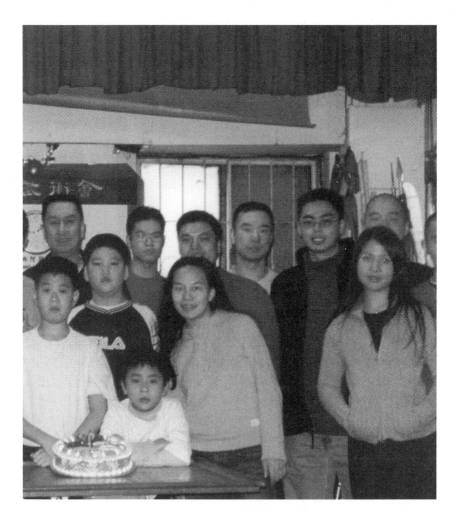

and integral part of our family, a link that will become stronger and stronger as each generation progresses. Kung Fu has now not only become a practice of a single person, but a tradition amongst everyone within the family.

It is often that those with foreign family ties will lose much of their culture and racial heritage when they travel to the United States. To a certain extent, I have fallen victim to this unfortunate side effect of separating from the homeland. However, my loss of culture would have been complete if it were not for my involvement Kung Fu. With the school located in the heart of Chinatown, New York, every visit of mine would be more than martial arts, but also a full immersion in the culture and customs of my ethnicity. Every corner would be full of much of what my heritage has come to stand for, and nearly all my knowledge of Chinese traditions have stemmed from what I have experienced in Chinatown and in Master Eng's school. Even my knowledge of martial arts is in itself an acknowledgement of my cultural heritage. Much of my identity as a person lies within my cultural and ethnical backgrounds and so much of who I am has stemmed from these cultural definitions that have been provided by my commitment to Kung Fu.

In being more than just an experience to be left behind, as with any other activity, martial arts is a mode of thinking, learning and for some, even a way of life. With such deep complexity as an abstract form, the teachings of Master Eng's have had powerful influences on every aspect of my life. Martial arts has had a profound effect on my expectations and patience with schoolwork and other activities. Starting Kung Fu at a young age, I learned very early that the greatest rewards in life are never direct or immediate. Such knowledge at an early age has taught me to have a great amount of patience and foresight in any endeavor I wish to accomplish, or any work that I attempt to create. Master Eng has taught me a strong discipline in order to achieve excellence in my martial arts and has no doubt shown me how to carry out any act to its completion. This no doubt has played one of the greatest parts in my accomplishments within any realm.

There are so many other aspects of myself that have been changed by my experiences with martial arts and Master Tak Wah Eng that it would be impossible to list, though it is very clear to me that nearly every facet of my personality has been shaped by this man and the revelation that is Kung Fu. Kung Fu has played so many parts in my life that it has become more than just a learning experience or a grand childhood memory. It has become a part of me, and doubtlessly, the part of me that I have come to love and respect the most.

Michael James Lee
Student of Sifu Tak Wah Eng
Tak Wah Eng Shaolin Kung Fu Club

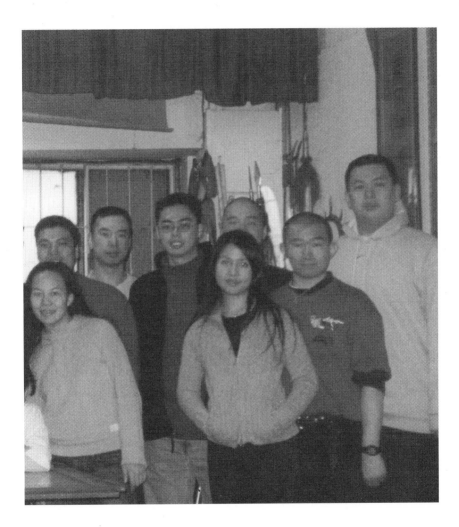

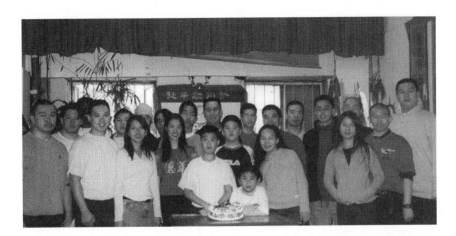

About the Author

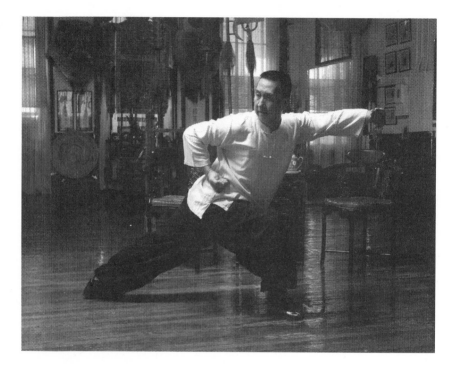

Master Tak Wah Eng began his martial arts training in Hong Kong during the tender age of ten. As many youths of this time he was filled with the stores of legendary heroes and of brave Shaolin warriors. His was initially exposed to Tai Chi and Southern Shaolin Kung Fu. He trained hard and was always eager to learn more.

During this time Hong Kong was still a rough town; life was hard and it offered few opportunities. His family then decided to try it out in America for a better life; and as with many immigrant families from Hong Kong they settled in New York's Chinatown.

In the late 1960s martial arts were all the rage and Kung Fu among the teenagers of Chinatown was no exception. Tak Wah Eng again wanted to pursue his martial arts training and his good fortune was to be introduced to Master Wai Hong of the Fu Jow Pai Kung Fu system. Under Wai Hong's tutelage Tak Wah Eng learned the finer points of the Tiger Claw System.

As luck would have it Master Eng was also privileged to meet and learn from Grandmaster Liu Ghi Rong of the Tai Kong Moon System, from the Hunan province. He was known as the "King of the Long Pole." Grandmaster Liu is now 89 years old and considered a living treasure in Chinese martial arts circles. Learning from Grandmaster Liu has given Master Eng greater insight into his own martial arts experience.

Many of Master Eng's students are well known. He has worked extensively in many action movies, acting as martial arts choreographer and trainer; and many have turned to him for his skill, guidance and wisdom. One such student is Russell Wong, who has trained hard with Master Tak Wah Eng for many years and has utilized his kung fu in various roles. Wong has starred in the television series "Vanishing Son" as well as the movie Romeo Must Die with Jet Li.

Master Tak Wah Eng's students are forever indebted to him for not only imparting his great skill, but also displaying the type of compassion and guidance that can only come from being Inside Kung Fu's 2001 "Instructor of the year".

佛

不生氣口訣

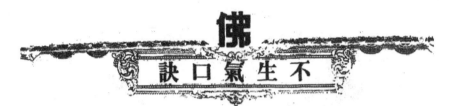

人生就像一場戲
因為有緣才相聚
相扶到老不容易
是否更該去珍惜
為了小事發脾氣
回頭想想又何必
別人生氣我不氣
氣出病來無人替
我若氣死誰如意
況且傷神又傷身
鄰居親朋不要比
兒孫瑣事由他去
吃苦享樂在一起
神仙羨慕好伴侶

吳氏姓名的　印